Gastrointesti... problems

YOUR QUESTIONS ANSWERED

For Elsevier

Commissioning Editor: Fiona Conn
Project Development Manager: Isobel Black
Project Manager: Nancy Arnott
Design Direction: George Ajayi
Illustration Manager: Bruce Hogarth

Gastrointestinal problems

YOUR QUESTIONS ANSWERED

John Hebden
BSc MD FRCP
Consultant Physician/Gastroenterologist
Sheffield Teaching Hospitals NHS Trust
Sheffield, UK

Mark Donnelly
FRCP
Consultant Physician/Gastroenterologist
Sheffield Teaching Hospitals NHS Trust
Sheffield, UK

Mark Rickets
BSc DGM DRCOG MRCGP
General Practitioner, The Nightingale
Practice, London, and Joint Head of GP
Development, City and Hackney PCT,
London, UK

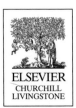

ELSEVIER
CHURCHILL
LIVINGSTONE

EDINBURGH LONDON NEW YORK OXFORD PHILADELPHIA ST LOUIS SYDNEY TORONTO 2006

ELSEVIER
CHURCHILL
LIVINGSTONE

First published 2006

ISBN-10: 0-443-07479-8
ISBN-13: 978-0-443-07479-0

British Library Cataloguing in Publication Data
A catalogue record for this book is available from the British Library

Library of Congress Cataloging in Publication Data
A catalog record for this book is available from the Library of Congress

Note
Knowledge and best practice in this field are constantly changing. As new research and experience broaden our knowledge, changes in practice, treatment and drug therapy may become necessary or appropriate. Readers are advised to check the most current information provided (i) on procedures featured or (ii) by the manufacturer of each product to be administered, to verify the recommended dose or formula, the method and duration of administration, and contraindications. It is the responsibility of the practitioner, relying on their own experience and knowledge of the patient, to make diagnoses, to determine dosages and the best treatment for each individual patient, and to take all appropriate safety precautions. To the fullest extent of the law, neither the publisher nor the authors assume any liability for any injury and/or damage to persons or property arising out of or related to any use of the material contained in this book.
The Publisher

ELSEVIER your source for books, journals and multimedia in the health sciences
www.elsevierhealth.com

The Publisher's policy is to use **paper manufactured from sustainable forests**

Printed in China

Contents

Preface

Perhaps gastroenterology is the most pervasive of all clinical specialties in medical practice. Certainly, people are frequently aware of symptoms arising from the gastrointestinal tract which, of course, are mostly self-managed in the community. These can range from an episode of diarrhoea and vomiting to concerns over diet and nutrition through to problems arising from more specific disease-based pathology. The book is structured so as to address the spectrum of issues that concern people and which form the questions presented to their attending clinicians.

This book is not just about the latest research into the subject. Rather, it seeks as its aim to help clinicians in their daily work by providing an evidence-based, expert opinion on the questions that patients pose in everyday clinical practice. It should also readily support decision making and act as a resource for professionals from all backgrounds (in practice and in training) and for patients with some pre-existing specialist knowledge to aid them in making the best possible decisions about their management.

Questions that range from explaining the new and esoteric to others which challenge time-honoured practice are posed, as well as addressing the sorts of problems that routinely face a GP, for instance, questions that they would want to discuss with a specialist colleague.

The chapters are presented starting with the mouth and working through the gastrointestinal system southwards, with various stops along the way to consider disorders affecting the liver, other related organs and extra-GI manifestations of gastrointestinal disease. The book continues with consideration of nutrition and obesity, screening and surveillance, investigations and further review of drug treatments. It finishes with the presentation of useful addresses, websites and journals which will point the enthusiast (both lay and professional) to sources of further reading.

The content of this book is not intended to be an exhaustive treatise on all aspects of gastroenterology since a subject as large as this can generate much longer tomes. However, we wanted to cover important issues succinctly, in a way that allows easy access to the information, and thereby produce a book that becomes a valued resource for those who use it.

JH
MD
MR

How to use this book

The *Your Questions Answered* series aims to meet the information needs of GPs and other primary care professionals who care for patients with chronic conditions. It is designed to help them work with patients and their families, providing effective, evidence-based care and management.

The books are in an accessible question and answer format, with detailed contents lists at the beginning of every chapter and a complete index to help find specific information.

ICONS

Icons are used in the book to identify particular types of information:

 highlights information important to clinical practice

 highlights side-effect information.

PATIENT QUESTIONS

At the end of relevant chapters there are sections of frequently asked patient questions, with easy-to-understand answers aimed at the non-medical reader. These questions are also listed at the end of the book.

The mouth and disorders of swallowing

1

1.1 What are the causes of a dry mouth?

A dry mouth (xerostomia) may be due to destruction/atrophy of the salivary glands, or secondary to medications.

Sjögren's syndrome, characterised by dry mouth, dry eyes (keratoconjunctivitis sicca) and arthritis, is due to an autoimmune destruction of the salivary glands. It may be a primary disorder, or secondary when it is associated with connective tissue disease (e.g. systemic lupus erythematosus, rheumatoid arthritis).

Medications causing a dry mouth include anticholinergics, tricyclic antidepressants, anti-Parkinsonian medication and diuretics.

1.2 How do you treat a dry mouth?

After investigating the underlying cause, symptomatic relief may be gained by encouraging regular sips of water, sucking mints or chewing gum. Artificial saliva (sodium carboxymethyl cellulose) may be required, and the cholinergics, pilocarpine and bethanechol, may be used.

1.3 What are the causes of glossitis?

Glossitis – inflammation of the tongue – results in erythema and atrophy of the papillae which at its most severe may result in a smooth, red 'beefy' tongue. Deficiencies in iron, vitamin B – including vitamins B2 (riboflavin), B3 (niacin), B6 (pyridoxine) and B12 (cobalamin) – and folic acid may all result in atrophic glossitis. Other causes include chemical irritants, amyloidosis, sarcoidosis and, naturally, pernicious anaemia.

1.4 What is black hairy tongue?

Black hairy tongue is the result of pigment deposition in elongated papillae and is commonly seen in chronic smokers and after antibiotic treatment. Treatment is improved attention to oral hygiene.

1.5 What is a geographical tongue, and what is its management?

Geographical tongue is a common (4% of the population) condition, the map-like appearance being caused by migratory patchy loss of filiform papillae. The condition is entirely benign and self-limiting and has no known association with serious underlying disease. Treatment is improved oral hygiene and may be helped by regular use of mouthwashes.

1.6 What causes aphthous ulcers?

These painful, shallow ulcers, covered in a yellow–white slough with surrounding erythema, are very common.

The aetiology is probably immunological and stress can precipitate them, although local physical trauma may also produce ulcers in susceptible individuals. Most are not associated with any underlying disease although identical lesions can occur more commonly in people with inflammatory bowel disease, coeliac disease, Behçet's syndrome, haematinic deficiencies and food sensitivities.

> If aphthous ulcers appear on keratinised mucosa (e.g. hard palate, posterior tongue), the cause may be herpes simplex infection. Healing occurs spontaneously over 1–2 weeks but frequent aciclovir use may accelerate resolution. More commonly (25% of the population), they appear on unkeratinised mucosa (e.g. labial and buccal mucosa) and are idiopathic.

1.7 What is dysphagia?

From the Greek, *phagia* (to eat) and *dys* (difficulty), this means the sensation of food (or fluids) 'sticking' between the mouth and stomach. It usually indicates organic disease and should always be investigated urgently (indeed, it is one of the alarm symptoms for upper gastrointestinal malignancy). Causes are many, and can be divided into oropharyngeal and oesophageal (*Box 1.1*).

1.8 What is odynophagia?

Odynophagia – pain on swallowing – indicates severe inflammation, for example due to infectious oesophagitis (Candida, cytomegalovirus) or severe ulcerative peptic oesophagitis. Rarely, patients with carcinoma may present with odynophagia without coexisting dysphagia. The occurrence of both symptoms together, especially with associated weight loss, is highly suggestive of oesophageal malignancy.

1.9 What is globus?

Globus is a tight feeling or lump in the throat, not related to swallowing. It is very common; almost half the population can experience this at some time, but it is especially frequent in middle-aged females. Globus is present between meals (contrast to odynophagia and dysphagia, which are not present during this time).

OESOPHAGEAL CANCER

1.10 What are the different types and causation of oesophageal carcinoma?

There are two different types of oesophageal carcinoma: squamous cell carcinoma and adenocarcinoma.

BOX 1.1 Causes of dysphagia

Oropharyngeal
- Neuromuscular, e.g. cerebrovascular accident, motor neurone disease
- Mechanical obstruction, e.g. cervical osteophyte
- Muscle disease, e.g. myasthenia gravis
- Others, e.g. Sjögren's syndrome

Oesophageal
- Mechanical obstruction, e.g. peptic strictures, webs and rings (Schatzki, *see Q 1.24*), neoplasm
- Dysmotility, e.g. achalasia
- Miscellaneous, e.g. reflux disease

Squamous cell carcinomas

Squamous cell carcinomas have traditionally been more common and occur in the mid or upper oesophagus. There is wide geographical variation in incidence, with pockets of very high incidence in northern Iran and southern Turkey. The explanation for this may be dietary (e.g. the ingestion of very hot liquids). Other recognised risk factors include smoking and chronic excessive alcohol intake.

Patients with achalasia (*see Q 1.18*) have an increased risk of squamous carcinoma (over 100-fold increased risk compared to unaffected individuals), as do patients with caustic strictures due to accidental or deliberate ingestion of such chemicals. Tylosis (characterised by hyperkeratosis of the palms and soles) and Patterson–Kelly syndrome (characterised by iron deficiency anaemia, spoon-shaped nails and oesophageal web) are other rare associations.

Adenocarcinoma

The main risk for adenocarcinoma appears to be acid reflux disease with the subsequent formation of Barrett's oesophagus (*see Q 2.36*). Barrett's confers an annual risk of developing cancer of 0.5–1.0% per annum, i.e. a 30- to 60-fold increase compared to the general population. Particular factors in Barrett's patients that offer additional risk appear to be a long segment (>5 cm), the presence of an ulcer in that segment, male sex, high body mass index and smoking (Lagegren et al 1999).

1.11 How common is oesophageal cancer?

The incidence of squamous cell carcinoma (SCC) and adenocarcinoma combined is 3–4:100 000. Men are affected more than women (3:1) and the median age of presentation is late sixties. Geographical variation in incidence is striking. Worldwide, SCC remains the commonest type; however, in the West, SCC has been overtaken by adenocarcinoma, which has risen fivefold in the last 30 years (Devesa et al 1998).

1.12 How does oesophageal cancer present?

Dysphagia (*see Q 1.7*) is the commonest symptom (90%), followed by odynophagia (*see Q 1.8*) (50%). Up to three-quarters of patients also have anorexia and weight loss at presentation. Patients may also present with vocal cord paralysis (recurrent laryngeal nerve involvement) and pain radiating to the back (implies mediastinal invasion); additionally, oesophago-tracheal fistulation with associated aspiration can occur (usually in squamous tumours). Haematemesis is a relatively unusual presentation but may be catastrophic and fatal if due to an oesophago-aortic fistula. Patients may develop pulmonary, brain, bone and liver metastases.

1.13 How should oesophageal cancer be investigated?

Gastroscopy (*see Q 13.7*) is the investigation of choice. Barium studies are now not used routinely but may be used as an adjunct, especially in particularly proximal or tight strictures. Once diagnosis is confirmed histologically and the patient deemed fit for oesophagectomy (tests of which may include assessment of cardiac and respiratory function with, for example, pulmonary function testing), the tumour must then be staged to guide optimal therapy.

1.14 How is oesophageal malignancy staged?

Modalities used in the staging of oesophageal malignancy include CT scanning, endoscopic ultrasound, positron emission tomography and laparoscopy (*Box 1.2*).

BOX 1.2 Modalities and their purpose in the staging of oesophageal malignancy

Modality	Purpose
CT scanning	Distant metastases, especially lung and liver
Endoscopic ultrasound	Tumour and local lymph node stage
Positron emission tomography	Distant metastases, especially lymph node and bone
Laparoscopy	Peritoneal disease in distal or junctional tumours

BOX 1.3 **Staging of oesophageal malignancy**

Stage	Definition
Tumour	
T0	No evidence of primary tumour
T1	Tumour invades lamina propria or submucosa
T2	Tumour invades muscularis mucosa
T3	Tumour invades adventitia
T4	Tumour invades adjacent structures
Nodes	
N0	No nodal metastasis
N1	Regional lymph node metastases
Distant metastases	
M0	No distant metastases
M1	Distant metastases

TABLE 1.1 American Joint Committee on Cancer (AJCC) tumour staging and recommended therapies

AJCC stage	TNM classification	Therapies
Stage 0	T0, N0, M0	Surgery or endoscopic mucosal resection
Stage I	T1, N0, M0	Surgery or endoscopic mucosal resection
Stage IIA	T2 or T3, N0, M0	Surgery with neoadjuvant chemotherapy
Stage IIB	T1 or T2, N1, M0	Surgery with neoadjuvant chemotherapy
Stage III	T3, N1 or T4, any N, M0	Surgery for T3 lesions with chemotherapy; palliation/chemotherapy alone for T4
Stage IV	Any T/N, M1	Palliation

At presentation, most patients have a T3 tumour (*Box 1.3*) or more; it is at this stage that lymph node metastases (or micrometastases) are almost universal. However, it is important to bear in mind that T3N0 staged tumours or those at a lower stage are potentially curable.

1.15 What treatment modalities are available?

Treatment depends on stage (*Table 1.1*). Surgical resection with neoadjuvant chemotherapy is currently thought to be the best therapy for those with potentially curable disease (Kelsen et al 1998). This is major surgery and there is no place for palliative oesophagectomy in those known to have incurable disease.

Palliation can involve both local and systemic treatments:
■ local therapies include stent insertion (with subsequent re-stenting or thermal ablation if the stent occludes), laser ablation and radiotherapy
■ systemic therapy comprises cisplatin-based chemotherapy.

1.16 What is the prognosis in oesophageal cancer?

Unfortunately, most patients present with incurable disease, with less than 20% surviving a year or more; 50% have distant metastases at presentation.

As few as 20% of those deemed suitable for attempted surgical cure survive 3 or more years.

1.17 Does the cancer's histological type (i.e. squamous or adenocarcinoma) affect management?

Previously, management of the two histological types was different, with radiotherapy being favoured for SCCs and chemotherapy for adenocarcinomas – both with or without surgery. Most recent trials have recruited both SCCs and adenocarcinomas and the treatment for both types is now the same.

ACHALASIA

1.18 What is achalasia?

Achalasia is the commonest of the hypermotility syndromes affecting the oesophagus. The word means 'failure to relax' and the condition is characterised by incomplete relaxation of the lower oesophageal sphincter. Patients present with dysphagia, chest discomfort and (in time) weight loss. In severe or chronic cases, the presentation may sound worryingly like oesophageal cancer.

1.19 How common is achalasia?

The annual incidence is 0.5–1 per 100 000 of the population. Undiagnosed early or mild cases are probably more common.

1.20 How is achalasia diagnosed?

A history of chronic progressive dysphagia (*see* Q 1.7) with eventual weight loss suggests the diagnosis. In early cases, gastroscopy may appear entirely normal as there is no structural abnormality to impede passage of the endoscope. More chronic cases often have a hugely dilated oesophagus, full of food debris, giving a clue to the diagnosis.

Barium radiology can be very helpful, displaying the characteristic 'rat's tail' appearance at the lower oesophageal sphincter. The confirmatory test is oesophageal manometry (*see* Q 13.21) which shows typical features.

Many conditions, including oesophagogastric cancer, can mimic achalasia and it is important to bear this in mind when making the diagnosis. Moreover, achalasia has long been recognised as a risk factor for oesophageal carcinoma (Wychulis et al 1981).

1.21 How is achalasia treated?

Several treatment modalities are available, as summarised in *Table 1.2.* Specific pharmacological therapy, other than adequate acid suppression, has no place in the modern management of this condition in those who are otherwise fit and willing to undergo the procedures outlined in *Table 1.2.*

In practice, treatment is tailored to the individual patient's circumstances. A frail elderly patient, unfit for surgery, in whom postdilatation oesophageal perforation would almost certainly be fatal, may be suited to repeated botulinum toxin injection. On the other hand, a younger fitter patient, unprepared to accept the small risk of perforation accompanying pneumatic dilatation may opt for laparoscopic myotomy. Often one or two attempts at pneumatic dilatation are made followed by surgery if these fail. The advent of laparoscopic as opposed to open surgery has greatly changed this aspect of management.

1.22 What complications can occur in achalasia?

Apart from the increased risk of carcinoma, patients may become malnourished and have recurrent aspiration pneumonia if untreated.

1.23 Are there any other types of oesophageal dysmotility?

There are other types of oesophageal dysmotility:

- *Hypermotile* problems vary from minor manometric abnormalities to severely symptomatic spastic incoordination (such as 'corkscrew oesophagus'). Treatment rests on ensuring adequate acid suppression, and the use of nitrates, tricyclic antidepressants and calcium channel blockers (particularly diltiazem). Manometry may guide endoscopic therapy (dilatation or botulinum toxin injection) in selected cases.
- *Hypomotile* problems are most often associated with systemic disease such as scleroderma or diabetes mellitus. Adequate acid suppression is the cornerstone of management.

WEBS AND RINGS

1.24 What is a Schatzki ring?

This is a common finding (6–14% of patients undergoing routine endoscopy) and a common entry in endoscopy reports. It consists of a thin membrane encircling the lumen occurring at the squamocolumnar junction.

TABLE 1.2 Treatment modalities in achalasia

	Initial response	Long-term response	Complications	Advantages	Disadvantages
Botulinum toxin injection	90% at 1 month	60% at 1 year	Mild and infrequent	Well tolerated and safe	Poor longer term outcome
Pneumatic dilatation	75% at 1 year	60% at 5 years	3–5% perforation	Fair long-term response	Perforation a concern
Open surgical myotomy	>90% at 1 year	>75% at 20 years	10% dysphagia, 10% reflux; <2% mortality	Best long-term response	Needs thoracotomy
Laparoscopic myotomy	>90% at 1 year	85% at 5 years	10% reflux	Avoids thoracotomy with comparable long-term results to open procedure	Long-term outcome unknown

These rings are probably congenital but may be related to acid reflux. Usually asymptomatic, they can cause acute food bolus obstruction and may need (even repeated) dilatation.

1.25 What are oesophageal webs?

These thin horizontal membranes are found more proximally. They start anteriorly and never completely encircle the lumen. They rarely cause symptoms but, if dysphagia does occur, treatment is simple dilatation, often achieved in the process of endoscopic intubation itself.

Although there is an association with Patterson–Kelly syndrome (iron deficiency anaemia and increased risk of oesophageal squamous carcinoma), such cases are rare.

PATIENT QUESTIONS

1.26 I get really painful aphthous ulcers. What are the best treatments?

Oral antiseptic mouth rinses (e.g. chlorhexidine) are known to reduce the severity of each episode of ulceration, but do not affect the incidence of ulceration.

Less good evidence exists regarding the usefulness of topical corticosteroids (e.g. Adcortyl in Orabase) but may be worth trying to reduce the length and severity of ulceration.

Avoidance of precipitating factors is clearly useful in management. For instance:

■ ensuring properly fitting dentures and addressing dental problems
■ reducing chronic stress and fatigue (often reported by patients as provoking development of ulcers).

Many 'over the counter' preparations exist that are claimed to be beneficial in management. Limited evidence exists to objectively support their usefulness. However, many patients report they do help ease symptoms and may be worth trying.

1.27 Some people say I have unspeakably bad halitosis. Should I see a doctor or a dentist?

Most halitosis or 'bad breath' is usually due to inadequate oral hygiene. Other contributing factors include smoking, dietary habits and excess alcohol. General oral hygiene methods usually result in improvement including regular brushing, flossing, tongue scraping and regular mouthwash use. Rarely, halitosis can indicate an underlying gastrointestinal disorder such as small bowel bacterial overgrowth.

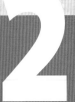

Dyspepsia and gastro-oesophageal reflux disease

2

PQ PATIENT QUESTIONS

DYSPEPSIA

2.1 What is dyspepsia?

Dyspepsia is a symptom. Although most patients who present with dyspepsia-like symptoms have no identifiable organic disease, others will have peptic ulcer disease, gastro-oesophageal reflux disease (GORD; *see Q 3.18*) and gastric carcinoma. Endoscopy might be regarded as the ideal initial investigation in dyspeptic patients; however, it is invasive, expensive and demand continues to rise year on year and outstrip supply. In the last few years research has focused on the idea of 'test and treat', i.e. test for *Helicobacter pylori* and treat (eradicate) if present, and reserve endoscopy for those aged 55 years and older, and those with persistent symptoms after eradication therapy. Any patient with alarm symptoms (anorexia, loss of weight, anaemia, mass, vomiting, haematemesis, dysphagia) should have an urgent endoscopy.

2.2 Can we define dyspepsia?

The most widely accepted definition of dyspepsia was described by a Rome working party in 1991 (Tally et al 1991). It defined dyspepsia as 'pain or discomfort centred in the upper abdomen'. Importantly, this definition excludes those patients with predominant reflux symptoms (acid regurgitation and heartburn) who should be regarded as suffering from GORD. An updated definition by the same working group defines 'centred' as meaning in or around the midline (Tally et al 1999).

2.3 What do the terms 'reflux-like dyspepsia', 'ulcer-like dyspepsia', 'dysmotility-like dyspepsia' and 'unspecified dyspepsia' mean?

These definitions were originally proposed as a means of subgrouping patients with dyspepsia according to their predominant symptoms, so as to reflect the most likely underlying pathology. In practice, however, these subgroupings are not clinically useful, with the exception of 'reflux-like dyspepsia', since they often overlap and lack predictive value for underlying disease. The more recent Rome criteria exclude 'reflux-like dyspepsia' from the definition of dyspepsia, with such patients considered as having GORD.

2.4 What is 'non-ulcer' or 'functional' dyspepsia?

The previous definitions of dyspepsia were based on symptoms alone. If investigated, a proportion of dyspeptic patients will be found to have peptic ulcer disease, reflux oesophagitis or other pathology. 'Non-ulcer' or 'functional' dyspepsia defines those patients with dyspepsia who do not have identifiable organic disease (i.e. those with a normal endoscopy ± normal blood tests).

2.5 How common is dyspepsia?

Dyspepsia is extremely common, with a prevalence of 25–40%. The wide variation probably reflects differences in populations and definitions. Only about 10% seek medical advice, comprising approximately 2–3% of all general practice consultations. About a fifth of these are referred to a specialist.

2.6 What is the prevalence of organic disease in patients with dyspepsia?

More than 50% of patients with dyspepsia who undergo endoscopy have normal findings (i.e. 'non-ulcer' or 'functional' dyspepsia). The other causes are peptic ulcer disease (20%), gastro-oesophageal reflux (20%) and gastric carcinoma (<2%). It should be noted, however, that many studies included patients with predominant gastro-oesophageal reflux symptoms, who would now be excluded from the 'dyspepsia' definition, thereby artificially elevating the proportion found to have GORD (Tally et al 1998a).

2.7 What are the most useful questions to ask when taking a history from someone with pain arising from the upper gastrointestinal tract?

In practice, the presentation of symptoms is often non-specific. This makes diagnosis difficult if working from history alone. However, the authors feel the following points are helpful in the development of a differential diagnosis in a patient who presents with pain thought to be arising from the upper gastrointestinal tract:

■ Epigastric pain that comes on during the night and is eased with the eating of food suggests a duodenal origin.
■ Epigastric pain that develops during the course of a meal suggests a gastric origin.
■ Epigastric pain that comes on some 30–60 minutes after a meal suggests pathology arising from the upper small bowel (e.g. Crohn's disease).
■ Pain which radiates from the epigastrium straight through into the back and is associated with weight loss suggests a pancreatic origin.
■ Pain radiating from the epigastrium retrosternally suggests oesophageal reflux.

2.8 How common is *Helicobacter pylori* infection?

Prevalence of *H. pylori* in many developed countries is higher in individuals born before 1950 (50–80%) compared with people born more recently (<20%). Lower social class is also associated with higher prevalence.

Infection is thought to occur primarily during childhood rather than throughout adult life.

2.9 How is *Helicobacter pylori* infection transmitted?

Overcrowded living conditions, especially when associated with poverty during childhood, are associated with a high level of transmission of *H. pylori* infection. Spread is presumed to be faecal–oral or oro–oral on the background of relatively poor sanitation. Close human adult contact in the presence of Western world standards of hygiene does not appear to lead to spread of infection.

Individuals suffering from *H. pylori* are highly unlikely to pass on the infection, even to a spouse.

2.10 What gastrointestinal tract diseases are associated with *Helicobacter pylori* infection?

The histological hallmark of Helicobacter infection is chronic gastritis. Other definite associations are duodenal ulcer disease, most gastric ulcers and MALToma (mucosal-associated lymphoid tissue tumour).

There is a strong association between Helicobacter infection and classic distal, antral gastric carcinoma. The association is not a simple one, however. The incidence of this disease has fallen in parallel with the decrease in the incidence of Helicobacter infection in the West and yet the overwhelming majority of patients with Helicobacter infection will not develop this tumour. Whether a particular individual develops no disease, gastritis, duodenal ulcer or gastric cancer depends on a host of factors including type and virulence of the infecting organism, age at infection, and genetic and environmental influences in the susceptible individual. Opinion varies as to whether Helicobacter should always be eradicated as a matter of course whenever it is detected and whether large resources should be devoted towards the development of an effective vaccine.

Although *H. pylori* has a causative role in gastric carcinoma, most infected people do not develop the disease, and the efficacy of successful eradication eliminating the risk of developing gastric carcinoma is unproven. However, it is the authors' practice to eradicate *H. pylori* infection if detected.

2.11 What is the best treatment for dyspepsia?

Most patients will present and be treated in general practice. The National Institute for Health and Clinical Excellence (NICE) have recently issued their guidelines on the management of dyspepsia (NICE 2004; *Fig. 2.1*). In summary these suggest:

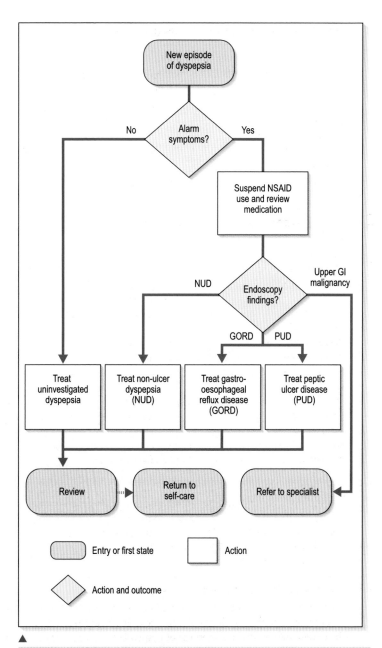

Fig. 2.1 Referral criteria and subsequent management of dyspepsia. (Reproduced with permission from the National Institute for Health and Clinical Excellence 2004.)

1. If, at any age, a patient has alarm symptoms, e.g. chronic gastrointestinal bleeding, anaemia, epigastric mass, persistent vomiting, progressive unintentional weight loss, suspicious barium meal or dysphagia, they should be referred urgently to secondary care (to be seen within 2 weeks). An acute gastrointestinal bleed demands immediate referral. At the time of referral, medications should be reviewed for possible precipitants of dyspepsia, e.g. calcium channel antagonists, nitrates, theophyllines, bisphosphonates, steroids and non-steroidal anti-inflammatory drugs (NSAIDs). Treatment thereafter is dependent on endoscopy findings, as for gastrointestinal malignancy, reflux disease, peptic ulcer disease or non-ulcer dyspepsia.

2. If there are no alarm symptoms, routine endoscopic investigation is not necessary. Over the age of 55, however, consider endoscopy when symptoms persist despite *H. pylori* testing [and eradication] or persist despite acid-suppressing therapy, and when patients have a history of previous gastric ulcer or surgery, a continuing need for NSAID therapy or a raised risk of gastric cancer or anxiety about cancer.

3. Patients who do not need referral for endoscopy (i.e. uninvestigated dyspepsia) should first have their medications reviewed for possible precipitants (see step 1 above), and be given lifestyle advice (healthy eating, weight reduction, smoking cessation, over-the-counter antacids). If there is no response or a relapse to this intervention, either: (a) treat with full-dose proton pump inhibitor (PPI) for 1 month, or (b) test (C13 urea breath test [C13UBT]/stool antigen/laboratory-based serology) and treat (PPI + amoxicillin + clarithromycin 500 mg, or PPI + metronidazole + clarithromycin 250 mg). If either (a) or (b) does not work, try the other. If both (a) and (b) are not successful, try a histamine type 2 receptor antagonist (H2RA) or a prokinetic (e.g. metoclopramide or domperidone) for 1 month. If (a) or (b) is successful but then symptoms recur, or there is a response to the H2RA/prokinetic, use low-dose treatment as required. If there is no response to this sequence, consider referral to a specialist for a second opinion.

2.12 What is the rationale behind 'test and treat' for dyspepsia?

The rationale behind testing for *H. pylori* and treating if present, rather than performing a gastroscopy, is based on:

- ■ *H. pylori* positive individuals having a higher prevalence of peptic ulcer disease (curable by eradication)
- ■ *H. pylori* negative individuals having either non-ulcer dyspepsia or gastro-oesophageal reflux disease, both of which are treated symptomatically
- ■ the risk of missing cancer in uncomplicated dyspepsia under the age of 55 years being extremely small.

A study from Glasgow looked at 327 consecutive patients referred for investigation of uncomplicated dyspepsia, with a mean age of 37 years (range 15–77 years). All patients had a C14 urea breath test and gastroscopy. Almost 60% were *H. pylori* positive, and in this group 40% had duodenal ulcer disease and 13% had gastric ulcers. In the group testing negative, duodenal ulcers were found in just 2% and gastric ulcers in 3%, with 17% having oesophagitis (McColl et al 1997).

A retrospective study from Gloucester reported on 319 gastric carcinomas diagnosed over a 6-year period. Of these, just 25 (7.8%) occurred in patients under 55 years of age, and 24 of the 25 had alarm symptoms (Christie et al 1997).

Tests for the detection of *H. pylori* are outlined in *Table 13.1*.

2.13 What is the cause of 'non-ulcer' or 'functional' dyspepsia?

The cause of functional dyspepsia is unknown. It is likely to be multifactorial, and as such it is not surprising that response to specific treatments is disappointing. Abnormalities of visceral perception, gastric emptying and gastric acid secretion have all been implicated.

2.14 Is *Helicobacter pylori* associated with 'non-ulcer' or 'functional' dyspepsia?

If *H. pylori* plays a role in functional dyspepsia, one would expect the prevalence to be higher in this group of patients compared to asymptomatic individuals. Data from individual studies are conflicting, but a meta-analysis of 23 observational studies showed that 55% of non-ulcer dyspeptic patients harboured *H. pylori* compared to 40% of controls, giving an odds ratio of 1.6 (95% CI, 1.4–1.8), $p < 0.001$ (Jaakkimainen et al 1999).

2.15 Should *Helicobacter pylori* be eradicated in patients with non-ulcer dyspepsia?

The small but significantly increased prevalence of Helicobacter in patients with non-ulcer dyspepsia suggests that it may play a role in some patients' symptoms. If so, eradication should result in symptom improvement (Drugs and Therapeutics Bulletin 2002). Again, individual trials give conflicting data.

There have been three published systematic reviews of data from randomised, placebo-controlled trials of eradication therapy in non-ulcer dyspepsia (Danesh et al 2000, Moayyedi et al 2000, Laine et al 2001). Two of these reviews showed no significant benefit, but the largest review collating data from nine trials involving over 2500 patients showed a small but significant reduction of 9% in dyspeptic symptoms in those receiving eradication therapy (Moayyedi et al 2000).

2.16 What is the best treatment for 'non-ulcer' or 'functional' dyspepsia?

'Non-ulcer' or 'functional' dyspepsia necessitates a negative gastroscopy for diagnosis. Many patients with uninvestigated dyspepsia will turn out to have functional dyspepsia if undergoing endoscopy, but this group of uninvestigated patients may also have gastric and duodenal ulcers and reflux disease.

- *Antacids* – Antacids do not appear to be helpful (Nyren et al 1986).
- *Histamine type 2 receptor antagonists (H2RAs)* – H2RAs are probably of no benefit either. Some studies have shown modest benefit, but this may be because the groups contained patients with reflux disease, and these patients would be expected to benefit from H2RA treatment.
- *Proton pump inhibitors (PPIs)* – PPIs appear to have a small but significant beneficial effect. In a 4-week, double-blind, randomised controlled trial in over 1200 patients with functional dyspepsia, resolution of symptoms was achieved in 38% on omeprazole 20 mg, 36% on omeprazole 10 mg and 28% on placebo (Tally et al 1998b). Subgroup analysis showed that the benefit occurred in those with ulcer-like or reflux-like functional dyspepsia, rather than the dysmotility type.
- Eradication of *H. pylori* – *see Question 2.15*.

The NICE (2004) guidelines suggest:

1. If *H. pylori* positive, eradicate; if response, return to self-care.
2. If *H. pylori* negative, or relapse/no response to step 1, try a low-dose PPI or H2RA for 1 month. If helpful, use on an as-required basis.
3. If there is an inadequate response, consider referral to a specialist.

2.17 What is the best treatment for peptic (gastric and duodenal) ulcer disease?

A proportion of gastric and duodenal ulcers will end up being treated (blindly) as part of the algorithm of management of simple, uninvestigated dyspepsia (by trial of PPI, or test and treat strategies). Some will, however, be discovered at endoscopy.

Gastric ulcer (GU)

The NICE (2004) guidelines suggest:

1. Stop NSAIDs if used, and test for *H. pylori* (C13UBT/stool antigen/laboratory-based serology). If NSAID continuation is necessary, offer long-term gastric protection or substitute to a Cox-2 selective

NSAID. [*Note: These guidelines were compiled before the publication of recent evidence concerning the safety profile of this class of drug.*]

2. If *H. pylori* positive and no NSAIDs are implicated, eradicate and repeat endoscopy 6–8 weeks later. If *H. pylori* positive and the ulcer is associated with NSAID use, treat with full-dose PPI for 2 months before eradication therapy, and then repeat endoscopy 6–8 weeks later. Retest for *H. pylori* with C13UBT; if the test remains positive, select second line eradication therapy from the *British National Formulary*. If the retest is negative and the ulcer is healed, use low-dose treatment as required, with periodic review. If the retest is negative and the ulcer has not healed (i.e. the patient is still symptomatic), refer to a specialist in secondary care if not already under their follow-up.

3. If *H. pylori* negative, treat with full-dose PPI for 1 or 2 months then repeat endoscopy. If the ulcer is healed, use low-dose treatment as required, with periodic review. If the ulcer is not healed, refer to a specialist in secondary care if not already under their follow-up.

Duodenal ulcer (DU)

The NICE (2004) guidelines suggest:

1. Stop NSAIDs if used, and test for *H. pylori* (C13UBT/stool antigen/laboratory-based serology). If NSAID continuation is necessary, offer long-term gastric protection or substitute to a Cox-2 selective NSAID. [*Note: These guidelines were compiled before the publication of recent evidence concerning the safety profile of this class of drug.*]

2. If *H. pylori* positive and the ulcer is associated with NSAID use, treat with full-dose PPI for 2 months, then eradication therapy. If response, discharge to self-care. If relapse/no response, retest for *H. pylori* with C13UBT; if positive, select second line eradication therapy. If response, discharge to self-care. If no response, use low-dose treatment as required, with review annually. If no response, also exclude other causes of DU (surreptitious or inadvertent aspirin/NSAID use, Zollinger–Ellison syndrome, Crohn's disease, false-negative *H. pylori* test, malignancy).

3. If *H. pylori* positive and no NSAIDs are implicated, eradicate. If response, discharge to self-care. If relapse/no response, retest for *H. pylori* with C13UBT; if positive, use second line eradication therapy and continue as in step 2.

4. If *H. pylori* negative, treat with full-dose PPI for 1–2 months. If response, use low-dose treatment as required, with review annually. If no response to full-dose, or low-dose treatment as required, exclude other causes of DU.

GASTRO-OESOPHAGEAL REFLUX DISEASE

2.18 What is gastro-oesophageal reflux disease?

Gastro-oesophageal reflux occurs normally (physiologically) in all people. Gastro-oesophageal reflux disease (GORD) is any symptomatic condition or pathophysiological alteration resulting from episodes of gastro-oesophageal reflux. This is usually taken to be acid, but bile may also be responsible.

GORD results in a spectrum of disease:

■ reflux oesophagitis
■ non-erosive GORD
■ acid-sensitive oesophagus.

2.19 What is reflux oesophagitis?

Reflux oesophagitis represents the most extreme end of the spectrum and is characterised by typical endoscopic lesions which may be graded according to severity (e.g. Savary–Miller grades I–IV or the new Los Angeles classification grades A–D) (*Box 2.1*). Approximately 20–30% of patients with typical GORD have endoscopic oesophagitis.

BOX 2.1 Savary–Miller and Los Angeles grading of reflux oesophagitis

Savary–Miller classification (most commonly used in the UK)
■ Grade I: One or more non-confluent erosions
■ Grade II: Confluent but not circumferential erosions
■ Grade III: Circumferential erosive oesophagitis
■ Grade IV: Grade III plus ulceration, stricture formation or Barrett's oesophagus

Los Angeles classification
■ Grade A: One (or more) mucosal breaks no longer than 5 mm that do not extend between the tops of two mucosal folds
■ Grade B: One (or more) mucosal breaks more than 5 mm long that do not extend between the tops of two mucosal folds
■ Grade C: One (or more) mucosal breaks that are continuous between the tops of two or more mucosal folds but involve <75% of the circumference
■ Grade D: One (or more) mucosal breaks that involve at least 75% of the oesophageal circumference

NB: the Los Angeles classification does not consider strictures or Barrett's oesophagus.

2.20 What is non-erosive (endoscopy-negative) GORD?

This is where a patient with typical symptoms of reflux has a normal endoscopy, but 24-hour ambulatory oesophageal pH (*see Q 2.31*) shows prolonged exposure of the oesophagus to acid. The usual cut-off regarded as normal is a pH <4 for less than 4% of the 24-hour period. Anything above this is regarded as abnormal and demonstrative of GORD.

2.21 What is an 'acid-sensitive' oesophagus?

A few patients have classic reflux symptoms but a normal endoscopy, and 24-hour ambulatory oesophageal pH (*see Q 2.31*) falls within normal limits. In such people, however, there is a strong correlation between normal 'physiological' acid reflux episodes (arbitrarily healthy people are allowed to have a pH <4 for up to 4% of the time in the distal oesophagus) and their symptoms. This can also be demonstrated by a Bernstein test which involves infusing normal saline and hydrochloric acid alternately into the oesophagus (with the patient blinded) and monitoring their symptoms. Patients in whom physiological acid exposure results in typical reflux symptoms are said to have an acid-sensitive oesophagus (i.e. hypersensitive).

2.22 How common is GORD?

GORD is extremely common, as evidenced by PPI prescriptions. It is estimated that 4–7% of the population experience heartburn daily, and that 33–44% of the population experience heartburn monthly. The prevalence of endoscopic reflux oesophagitis is estimated at 2%, and autopsy studies show a prevalence of Barrett's oesophagus (extreme end of the reflux spectrum) of 1%.

GORD is becoming more common, rising exponentially over the last 30 years, in contrast to duodenal ulcer disease which is showing the reverse trend.

2.23 How well does the symptom of heartburn predict GORD?

Heartburn is poorly predictive of endoscopic oesophagitis, as evidenced by the fact that 70–80% of endoscopies will be normal. Twenty-four-hour oesophageal pH studies show that the frequency (not the severity) of heartburn correlates with the percentage of time that the distal oesophagus is exposed to acid (Joelsson & Johnsson 1989).

2.24 What causes GORD?

The barrier mechanism is complex and not completely understood. The two main mechanisms appear to be the lower oesophageal sphincter and the crural diaphragm. Transient lower oesophageal sphincter relaxations (TLESRs), which occur physiologically during belching, also appear to be important.

2.25 How does the lower oesophageal sphincter act as a barrier?

The lower oesophageal sphincter (LOS) maintains a resting tone of 10–30 mmHg, thereby preventing free reflux of stomach contents into the oesophagus. It is, however, in a dynamic state, with certain foods, sleep, gastric distension, hormones and some medications capable of altering its tone. Chocolate, caffeine, alcohol, fat and peppermint all decrease LOS tone. Beta-adrenergic agonists (e.g. salbutamol, nitrates, calcium antagonists and theophylline) also decrease LOS tone.

Twin studies suggest that there may also be a genetic predisposition to GORD.

Strain-induced reflux (e.g. coughing, bending) is rare unless the LOS pressure is <10 mmHg, and free reflux does not occur unless the LOS pressure is <4 mmHg. Only a minority of GORD patients, however, have a resting LOS pressure <10 mmHg. The majority must be susceptible during periodic decreases due to certain foods or drugs, or other phenomena such as TLESRs.

2.26 What is the significance of a hiatus hernia?

Hiatal hernias (i.e. herniation of a portion of the stomach above the crural diaphragm and into the chest) are seen frequently at endoscopy. Although not necessarily causing symptoms, they do play a part in GORD in some patients. They are not a prerequisite, however, since 50% of patients with GORD do not have a hiatus hernia.

The size of the hiatus hernia is important in strain-induced reflux. At any given LOS pressure, the larger the hiatus hernia, the greater the degree of reflux induced by straining (Sloan et al 1992).

2.27 What is the role of *Helicobacter pylori* in GORD?

Helicobacter pylori plays no role in the causation or cure of GORD.

Some earlier publications reported an increase in reflux symptoms following eradication of *H. pylori*, but other studies were contradictory. Theoretically it is appealing. *H. pylori* causes gastritis and a reduced acid output from the stomach. Eradication would resolve the gastritis and allow improved parietal (acid) cell function. A recent large meta-analysis, however, showed no increase in GORD symptoms following eradication of *H. pylori* (Moayyedi et al 2001).

2.28 If I am treating GORD with a proton pump inhibitor, should I eradicate *Helicobacter pylori*?

As mentioned in *Question 2.27*, some earlier publications reported an increase in GORD symptoms following eradication of *H. pylori*. It was therefore thought that GORD might respond better to acid-suppressing therapy in the presence of *H. pylori* infection. Against this is the fact that *H. pylori*-induced gastritis predisposes to gastric atrophy and the pathway leading to intestinal metaplasia, dysplasia and carcinoma. A study in the 1990s reported an increase in gastric atrophy in *H. pylori* positive GORD patients who were treated with a PPI compared to *H. pylori* positive GORD patients who had anti-reflux surgery. In other words, a PPI and *H. pylori* were synergistic in promoting gastric atrophy (Kuipers et al 1996). Other studies, however, have not supported these data (Lundell et al 1999).

It is the authors' opinion that *H. pylori* should be eradicated if found during the investigation of GORD for the following reasons:

- *H. pylori* and PPIs may promote gastric atrophy
- *H. pylori* is a class A carcinogen
- Why test for *H. pylori* if the intention is not to treat if present?

2.29 How should I manage GORD?

The history is usually sufficient to diagnose reflux disease and start treatment with antacids or acid-suppressing therapy. Many people have only mild or intermittent symptoms, and respond well to antacids, and to dietary and lifestyle modifications.

Diagnostic studies (gastroscopy, 24-hour oesophageal pH and manometry, etc.; *see Ch. 13*) are indicated when symptoms are:

- chronic
- refractory to treatment
- atypical
- associated with warning signs.

The usual first line investigation is a gastroscopy.

2.30 How sensitive is a gastroscopy in diagnosing GORD?

Only 20–30% of GORD patients will have erosive oesophagitis at gastroscopy. Around 70% of gastroscopies will be normal, indicating that the patient has non-erosive (endoscopy-negative) GORD, an acid-sensitive oesophagus or a different diagnosis (e.g. cardiac pain).

2.31 What is 24-hour ambulatory oesophageal pH?

Twenty-four-hour oesophageal pH monitoring represents the gold standard for detecting acid reflux disease, since reflux does not always cause macroscopic oesophagitis.

It involves placing (through the nostril) a thin catheter with a pH-sensitive probe at the distal end, 5 cm above the gastro-oesophageal junction. Data are then recorded over a 24-hour period. Arbitrarily, a cut-off value of pH <4 for less than 4% of the 24-hour period is regarded as normal (*Fig. 2.2*). Anything above this indicates significant acid reflux disease (*Fig. 2.3*).

2.32 How sensitive is 24-hour oesophageal pH monitoring if a patient is not getting symptoms every day?

The sensitivity of this test is positively correlated with the frequency of heartburn and acid regurgitation. Therefore, a false-negative result may occur in patients who are only experiencing intermittent symptoms (Joelsson & Johnsson 1989).

2.33 How should I treat GORD?

It is sensible to advise dietary and lifestyle measures. These include stopping smoking, losing weight if obese, reducing alcohol intake and avoiding large

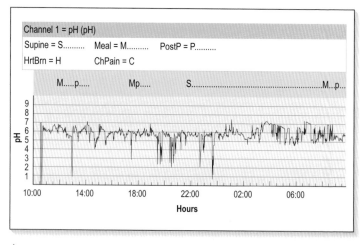

Fig. 2.2 Normal 24-hour oesophageal pH profile. Note occasional 'spikes' of acid into oesophagus that are quickly cleared with pH returning towards neutral. (Courtesy of Pat Vales, Gastrointestinal Physiology Department, Manchester Royal Infirmary, Manchester.)

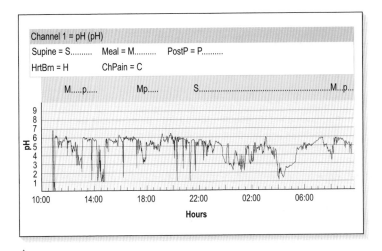

Channel 1 = pH (pH)

Supine = S.......... Meal = M.......... PostP = P.........

HrtBrn = H   ChPain = C

M.....p....   Mp.....   S...M..p...

Fig. 2.3 Abnormal 24-hour oesophageal pH profile. Note the prolonged dips in pH, with a marked dip between 0400h and 0530h during sleep.

meals before bed. Certain foods and drugs may precipitate symptoms. Chocolate, caffeine, alcohol, fat and peppermint relax the lower oesophageal sphincter, as do some drugs such as calcium antagonists and nitrates, and may contribute to reflux symptoms. Most of these measures, however, will not have major effects on those with moderate to severe GORD.

The majority of GORD patients with moderate to severe symptoms (and/or erosive oesophagitis) will require acid-suppressing treatment with H2RAs or PPIs. Treatment may follow a 'step-up' approach, starting with a H2RA and moving onto a PPI if necessary, or a 'step-down' approach. PPIs are vastly superior to H2RAs in both the relief of symptoms and the healing of endoscopic oesophagitis. Severe endoscopic oesophagitis demands a more aggressive approach than non-erosive (endoscopy-negative) reflux disease, since the former may result in stricture formation.

Recent guidelines have been produced by NICE (2004). In summary these suggest:

1. Uninvestigated 'reflux disease' should be managed in the same way as uninvestigated dyspepsia (*see* Q 2.11).
2. If endoscopy shows macroscopic oesophagitis, the patient should be treated with full-dose PPI for 1–2 months; if they respond, then step down to the lowest dose to control symptoms. If symptoms do not respond to full-dose PPI, the dose should be doubled for 1 month; if response is then achieved, again step down to the lowest dose to control

symptoms. If the patient did not respond to the double dose PPI, then a H2RA or prokinetic can be tried for 1 month. If responding, titrate down to the lowest dose that controls symptoms; if no response, consider referral to secondary care.

3. If endoscopy is negative (as in 70–80% of patients with reflux disease), the patient should have a trial of full-dose PPI. If they respond, reduce down to the lowest dose to control symptoms. If symptoms do not respond to full-dose PPI, try a H2RA or prokinetic for 1 month. If response is then achieved, titrate down to the lowest dose that controls symptoms; if no response, consider referral to secondary care.

2.34 Which proton pump inhibitor should I use to treat GORD?

There are currently five PPIs available: omeprazole, lansoprazole, rabeprazole, pantoprazole and esomeprazole. It is difficult to compare the different PPIs as treatment and maintenance doses differ. In general terms, milligram for milligram there is little or no difference between the different formulations. Choice will therefore be based largely on price.

Pantoprazole, by virtue of its metabolism, has no interaction with warfarin, and therefore is potentially useful in patients on multiple medications. Esomeprazole 40 mg has been shown (perhaps not surprisingly, given the higher milligram dosage) to be superior to lansoprazole 30 mg in the healing of endoscopic reflux oesophagitis, particularly the more severe end of the spectrum (Castell et al 2002).

 PPIs are very well tolerated. The most common side-effect is probably diarrhoea, which occurs in up to 5% of patients.

2.35 Which proton pump inhibitor should I use for maintenance?

Moderate to severe GORD should be regarded as a chronic disease, since 80% of patients have a relapse of their symptoms after cessation of treatment. Such patients are generally maintained on a low dose of a PPI. Again, milligram for milligram there is likely to be very little difference between the formulations. It is probably better to think of PPI dosage 10–20 mg as low dose, and PPI dosage 30–40 mg as high dose.

Recently, esomeprazole 20 mg has been shown to be superior to lansoprazole 15 mg in the maintenance of reflux oesophagitis, with the greatest difference seen with more severe disease (esomeprazole maintained 76% Los Angeles grade D oesophagitis (*see Box 2.1*) versus 50% maintained with lansoprazole) (Lauritsen et al 2003).

2.36 What is Barrett's oesophagus?

Barrett's oesophagus describes replacement of the normal squamous cell mucosal lining of the oesophagus by specialised columnar cell lining. This 'metaplastic' lining extends for a variable distance proximally from the gastro-oesophageal junction and is in contiguity with the gastric mucosa. Clinicians will normally diagnose Barrett's oesophagus if this lining extends for more than 3 cm; 'short-segment Barrett's oesophagus' refers to a length less than 3 cm. Autopsy studies suggest that Barrett's oesophagus of over 3 cm in length is present in approximately 1% of the population.

2.37 What causes Barrett's oesophagus?

Barrett's oesophagus is thought to result from excess acid reflux and is viewed as representing the most extreme end of the spectrum of acid reflux disease. Its prevalence is much higher in those with reflux symptoms, being present in approximately 10% of reflux sufferers. Short-segment Barrett's oesophagus is even more prevalent in this group of patients, being present in approximately 20%. It is not clear whether bile reflux has a role in its development.

2.38 What is the risk of developing oesophageal carcinoma in Barrett's oesophagus?

The risk of developing carcinoma is approximately 0.5–1% per annum (1 case per 100–200 patient years of follow-up), with reports ranging from 1 in 52 patient years of follow-up (approximately 2% per annum) to 1 in 441 patient years (approximately 0.2% per annum).

2.39 Should patients with Barrett's oesophagus undergo regular surveillance endoscopy?

The rationale behind surveillance endoscopy is that Barrett's is a significant risk factor for the development of oesophageal carcinoma, and that by detecting asymptomatic dysplastic change or early (curable) carcinoma, prognosis will be improved (*see also Q 12.21*). Most oesophageal carcinomas that are diagnosed following the development of dysphagia are inoperable (overall 5-year survival rate is just 5%).

Although the majority of gastroenterologists in the UK will enter patients into surveillance programmes, the evidence that this improves the survival of those who develop malignant transformation is controversial. There is some evidence that tumours are identified at an earlier stage, but as oesophageal carcinoma has such a universally poor prognosis, it is not certain whether such a strategy improves prognosis.

Surveillance gastroscopy is usually performed 1–2 yearly, although cost–benefit analysis suggests that 3 yearly is optimal. If low grade dysplasia is detected, the interval between endoscopic screening is shortened (e.g. 6 monthly). If high grade dysplasia is detected (and verified by a second pathologist), it is usual to advise/offer oesophagectomy, since coexistent carcinoma has been reported to be present in up to 50% of resected specimens.

2.40 Up to what age should surveillance of Barrett's oesophagus continue?

Surveillance is usually continued until the time at which the patient would not be considered fit enough to undergo oesophagectomy. It is important to appreciate that the time sequence for the development of dysplastic change thereafter, through to the development of asymptomatic carcinoma and then symptomatic carcinoma and death, is likely to be many years, and many elderly patients would want to take this into account before making a decision about treatment. In addition, the mortality from oesophagectomy is between 5 and 10%, and is associated with significant perioperative morbidity.

2.41 What are the treatment options and prognosis of oesophageal squamous cell carcinoma and oesophageal adenocarcinoma?

Oesophageal squamous cell carcinomas and adenocarcinomas are treated by surgical resection if staging (CT and/or endoscopic ultrasound) is favourable. Of the minority of patients that are suitable for surgical resection, those found to be node negative at histological examination have approximately 40% 5-year survival, whereas node-positive patients have a 15–20% 5-year survival.

Inoperable patients will be offered palliative stenting, laser therapy or radiotherapy.

 PATIENT QUESTIONS

2.42 I have heard that heartburn/reflux disease can cause oesophageal cancer. Is this true?

Yes, but the absolute risk is extremely small. In the USA, the prevalence of all tissue types of oesophageal cancer is around 3.3 per 100 000. Many people suffer from reflux disease (up to 20% will experience heartburn at some time), but very few people develop oesophageal carcinoma.

Evidence for reflux disease being a risk factor for the development of oesophageal carcinoma comes from a retrospective study in which patients with oesophageal squamous cell carcinoma and patients with oesophageal adenocarcinoma were asked about previous heartburn/reflux history. In those with severe heartburn for more than 20 years, the odds ratio was 43.5 for developing oesophageal adenocarcinoma compared to healthy controls, whereas the odds ratio for developing oesophageal squamous cell carcinoma was only 2 (thereby eliminating the potential recall bias of patients with cancer) (Lagergren et al 1999). Additionally it is believed that most oesophageal adenocarcinomas arise from Barrett's, which itself represents the more severe end of the spectrum of reflux disease.

2.43   My father died of oesophageal cancer. Is it inherited and should I be screened?

No. The cause of oesophageal carcinoma is multifactorial: Barrett's, smoking and alcohol are all associated. The influence of genetics (and therefore inheritance) is not thought to play any major role, and therefore there is no evidence that you will be at any particularly increased risk for the development of the disease, and as such you would not need to enter into any screening or surveillance programme.

2.44   I suffer from heartburn and need to take medicine (cimetidine, ranitidine [H2RAs], omeprazole, lansoprazole, pantoprazole, rabeprazole, esomeprazole [PPIs]) every day to keep my symptoms controlled. Will I come to any harm?

Whilst almost no drug is completely devoid of potential side-effects, these medicines (histamine type 2 receptor antagonists [H2RAs] and proton pump inhibitors [PPIs]) are very safe, even in long-term use.

The most commonly used drugs (after the over-the-counter antacids) to control reflux disease are the PPIs (the 'prazoles'). This drug class is one of the most commonly prescribed in the world, and data from long-term use (>10 years) show that they are very safe with no serious complications. The most common side-effect is diarrhoea, but this occurs in less than 5% of patients.

2.45   Does stress cause ulcers?

In extremely ill patients (e.g. with extensive burns or requiring intensive care), peptic ulcers – known as 'stress ulcers' – may occur. However, other forms of stress and anxiety do not cause peptic ulcer disease.

2.46   My symptoms of dyspepsia settled after *Helicobacter pylori* eradication therapy. Do I ever need to be tested again to see if it has come back?

H. pylori eradication therapy is highly successful, eradicating the bacteria in 85–90% of patients. If your dyspepsia was secondary to ulcer disease, your symptoms should disappear completely. Unless symptoms recur, routine testing for successful *H. pylori* eradication is not recommended.

2.47   Can I pass *Helicobacter pylori* on to other members of my family?

Infection is generally acquired in childhood. It is rare for adults to pass it on to other adults. The most important recognised factor in determining the risk of infection is the socioeconomic status of the family during childhood.

The exact mechanism for transmission remains uncertain and debate continues; therefore no clear guidance currently exists to answer this question.

Other upper gastrointestinal problems

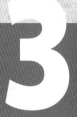

3

GALLSTONES

3.1 How common are gallstones?

Ten per cent of Western populations have gallstones. They are very rare in African and Asian populations although incidence is increasing in response to a change to Western diet and lifestyle. Native Americans have the highest incidence, linked to cholesterol supersaturation of bile.

> Asymptomatic gallstones are very common. The presence of gallstones on ultrasound scan does not automatically warrant referral for surgical opinion regarding possible laparoscopic surgery.

3.2 What are the different types of gallstones?

Gallstones are predominantly composed of cholesterol (commonest in Western populations); more rarely, they contain bilirubin (black pigment) or calcium bilirubinate (brown pigment).

3.3 What causes gallstones?

There are three major factors in gallstone formation:

- supersaturation of bile with cholesterol (increased bile cholesterol concentration compared to bile acid levels)
- the tendency of that cholesterol to aggregate (called 'nucleation')
- impaired gallbladder function with particular respect to inadequate contraction.

Infection may play a role in some cases by providing a nidus for nucleation, and incidence certainly increases with age (up to 20% of men and 35% of women have gallstones by age 75). Relatives of affected individuals have a two to four times increased risk of gallstones. Women are two to three times more likely to develop gallstones than men premenopausally; after the menopause, incidence rates level off between the sexes.

Obesity is also a risk factor. A linear relationship exists between body mass index (BMI) and gallstone development. Conversely, rapid weight loss is also associated, especially if achieved by surgical means, presumably because of an interruption in the normal enteropathic bile circulation. Total parenteral nutrition is also a risk factor.

Pregnancy is an association but 'fertility' per se appears to contribute little to overall risk.

Various drugs are associated with gallstone formation including oestrogens and clofibrate. High serum cholesterol is not associated but raised serum triglycerides are a risk factor. Finally, patients with terminal ileal disease and consequent excessive bile salt excretion (classically Crohn's disease) are also at increased risk of developing gallstones.

3.4 Are gallstones always symptomatic?

Seventy-five per cent of gallstones are asymptomatic. The commonest clinical presentation (20%) is of intermittent pain – biliary colic – caused by stones intermittently obstructing the cystic duct. This consists of epigastric or right upper quadrant pain lasting for hours with associated nausea: 30% of patients have only a single such attack, 6% per year develop further symptoms and 1% per year develop a serious complication (e.g. cholangitis; *see Q 3.6*). Ten per cent of patients with gallstones develop acute cholecystitis, caused by impaction of the stone in the cystic duct.

3.5 How does acute cholecystitis present?

Most patients have had preceding attacks of biliary colic. Acute cholecystitis is characterised by prolonged pain (>6 hours), together with vomiting and pyrexia. Half of such patients will resolve spontaneously in 7–10 days; 10% will develop a localised perforation if left untreated.

3.6 What are the complications of cholecystitis?

Choledocholithiasis (intermittent obstruction of the common bile duct) may lead to cholangitis (5% of all gallstone patients), characterised by Charcot's triad of pain, jaundice and fever. Untreated, this condition carries a high mortality rate.

Mirizzi's syndrome is the rare complication of a cystic duct stone causing common bile duct obstruction indirectly. Less than 0.1% of patients with gallstones develop gallbladder carcinoma resulting from chronic cholecystitis.

3.7 What other complications do gallstones cause?

Apart from the previously described biliary colic, cholecystitis, choledocholithiasis and cholangitis, most other complications are relatively rare. The exception is gallstone pancreatitis which occurs in 3–7% of patients with gallstones, causing 35% of acute pancreatitis. Men are more likely to be affected (although most cases are in women because of the higher incidence of gallstone formation premenopausally) and commoner with small stones (<5 mm diameter) which are able to pass through the common bile duct to be impacted at the ampulla, causing pancreatic duct obstruction and hence inflammation. Cholecystectomy with bile duct clearance prevents recurrence.

Other rare complications of gallstones include emphysematous cholecystitis (gallbladder wall infected by gas-forming organisms), cholecystoenteric fistula formation with subsequent gallstone ileus, Mirizzi's syndrome (*see Q 3.6*) and porcelain gallbladder (calcification due to chronic inflammation) with consequent carcinoma.

3.8   How are gallstones diagnosed?

Ultrasonography (US) is the mainstay of gallstone diagnosis. It is more than 95% accurate in detecting gallbladder stones >2 mm in size. US is less effective in diagnosing common bile duct (CBD) stones (50% accurate). Magnetic resonance imaging of the biliary tree (so-called MRCP – magnetic resonance cholangiopancreatography; *see Q 13.9*) is an accurate way of diagnosing CBD stones, replacing endoscopic retrograde cholangiopancreatography (ERCP; *see Q 13.8*) for this purpose, the latter being reserved for treating such stones. Endoscopic ultrasound (EUS; *see Q 13.10*) is an accurate diagnostic tool for gallstones but is relatively invasive and not widely available in the UK.

3.9   Are medical treatments effective?

Non-surgical treatment of gallstone disease has proved an elusive goal. Despite much endeavour, surgical treatment is still the much-preferred option. Oral bile acid dissolution therapy (with ursodeoxycholic or chenodeoxycholic acid) is reserved for small radiolucent stones and extracorporeal shock wave lithotripsy for larger stones (70–80% of patients are stone-free at 12 months). Both techniques are limited in availability.

Even if successfully treated, the underlying factors for gallstone formation are not, of course, resolved with either approach. The advent of (relatively non-invasive) laparoscopic cholecystectomy (*see Q 3.10*) has largely confined these medical approaches to a few specialist centres.

3.10   What surgical treatments are effective?

Laparoscopic cholecystectomy is now the gold standard for treatment of gallbladder stones. Length of stay, morbidity, postoperative complications and mortality are all reduced in expert hands. Conversion rate to open cholecystectomy is 5% or less and more likely in obese patients or those with a previous history of upper abdominal surgery and subsequent adhesion formation.

The timing of surgery can be difficult. A single attack of mild biliary colic in an otherwise fit and well young patient may reasonably lead directly to surgery. On the other hand, patients with co-morbidity may well best be suited to conservative management. When the avoidance of complications of gallstones (e.g. cholangitis, pancreatitis) becomes more important than preventing possible operative complication, surgery would seem necessary. There is a distinct trend towards operation during the first admission with acute cholecystitis rather than the former practice of initial conservative management followed by subsequent elective surgery (Lai et al 1998, Lo et al 1998). Nevertheless, the timing and even mode of surgery should be individualised for each patient (Papi et al 2004).

3.11 Do gallstones recur after surgery?

Postsurgical CBD stones may be the result of such stones overlooked at the time of surgery or, less likely (probably in 1% of such patients), stones forming de novo in the duct remnant.

3.12 What are the potential complications of gallstone surgery?

Overall, laparoscopic cholecystectomy is a safe operation with a mortality rate of 0.1% or less and a morbidity rate of around 5%. Apart from general complications such as infection (systemic or wound) and complications from general anaesthesia, bile duct injury is the most noteworthy perioperative complication, affecting up to 1% of cases. This seems to be decreasing in incidence as laparoscopic skills, training and equipment are improving.

Longer term specific complications from surgery include the postcholecystectomy syndrome – the persistence of gastrointestinal symptoms following surgery – occurring in 5–40% of patients. Characteristics and causes are manifold but include retained or recurrent stones, wound pain and the original cause for the symptoms being something other than gallstones. Patients may experience diarrhoea postcholecystectomy due to an alteration in the enterohepatic bile circulation.

The supposed link between cholecystectomy and the subsequent development of bowel cancer is unproven.

PANCREATITIS

3.13 What is pancreatitis?

This is inflammation of the pancreas. *Acutely*, this may involve other local structures or other organ systems. *Chronic* pancreatitis is characterised by fibrotic destruction of the pancreatic gland with subsequent loss of exocrine and endocrine function.

3.14 How common is acute pancreatitis?

Estimates vary from 20 to 40 per 100 000 of the population per year. This leads to over 100 000 admissions per year in the US with 2000+ deaths (Steinberg & Tenner 1994).

3.15 What causes acute pancreatitis?

The causes of acute pancreatitis, and their frequency, are outlined in *Box 3.1*.

3.16 Is acute pancreatitis dangerous?

The severity of acute pancreatitis is assessed using a series of clinical and laboratory parameters to achieve a score – such as that used by APACHE II or Glasgow/Ransom criteria. 'Severe' pancreatitis, as measured by these various scoring systems, carries a mortality rate approaching 60%. Most patients, however, do not present with severe disease. Overall mortality rate is 5–10%

3.17 How does acute pancreatitis present?

Abdominal pain radiating from the epigastrium through to the back, with vomiting, are the classical symptoms of acute pancreatitis. Jaundice (because of associated cholangitis) is unusual. On examination, abdominal tenderness is common, and bowel sounds may be diminished. In severe cases, cardiovascular collapse and peritonism may be present.

Diagnosis rests upon the typical clinical presentation accompanied by a threefold rise in serum pancreatic enzymes (typically amylase). There are often characteristic radiological findings on CT scanning.

3.18 How is acute pancreatitis treated?

Acute pancreatitis is a surgical/gastroenterological emergency. Care is most often supportive (fluid resuscitation, intravenous antibiotics, etc.). Surgery may be necessary in selected cases (e.g. tissue necrosis, abscess formation).

BOX 3.1 Causes and frequency of acute pancreatitis

Cause	Frequency (%)
Gallstones (more common in women)	30–50
Alcohol (more common in men)	10–40
Trauma (ERCP/blunt trauma, etc)	5
Idiopathic	15
Drugs (e.g. azathioprine, furosemide)	
Pancreas divisum (congenital anatomical variant)	
Hypertriglyceridaemia	All rare
Hypercalcaemia	
Viral (mumps, cytomegalovirus, etc.)	
Hereditary	

ERCP, endoscopic retrograde cholangiopancreatography.

Some centres perform emergency ERCP on patients suspected of having gallstone pancreatitis.

3.19 What are the complications of acute pancreatitis?

Most cases settle spontaneously with conservative measures. Complications include abscess and pseudocyst formation, pancreatic necrosis and fat necrosis.

3.20 How common is chronic pancreatitis?

This is rare (less than 5 per 100 000 of the population per annum) and is most commonly caused by chronic alcohol abuse. Other causes (e.g. hereditary, idiopathic and cystic fibrosis) are all relatively rare.

3.21 How does chronic pancreatitis present?

Chronic abdominal pain (again, epigastric with radiation to the back) is common, with or without exocrine (diarrhoea/malabsorption) or endocrine (diabetes) insufficiency. There may be typical radiological findings (calcification in a third on plain film or CT), and tests of exocrine function may be abnormal (e.g. low faecal elastase).

3.22 How is chronic pancreatitis treated?

The management of pain is the mainstay of therapy. Once specific causes have been excluded (e.g. pseudocyst formation, bile duct obstruction), analgesics should be prescribed and alcohol avoided. Referral to a specialist pain management service can be invaluable. There is variable evidence of the utility of decreasing intrapancreatic pressure with the use of enzyme supplements or endoscopic stenting, but the former strategy, in particular, is widely used. In severe cases with intractable pain, coeliac plexus blockade (using radiological or endosonographic guidance) or even surgical pancreatectomy may be indicated.

3.23 How can pancreatitis be prevented?

Dealing with the underlying cause (avoidance of alcohol, gallstone surgery) is essential to avoid recurrent attacks of acute pancreatitis. The same measures may help ameliorate chronic pancreatitis.

PANCREATIC CANCER

3.24 How common is pancreatic cancer?

Incidence is increasing worldwide (5–10 per 100 000 of the population), with a preponderance in males (1.3:1).

3.25 What causes pancreatic cancer?

Usually an adenocarcinoma in nature, risk factors include age, male sex, smoking, chronic pancreatitis, diabetes and hereditary pancreatitis. There are possible links to excess dietary animal fat and protein. Conversely, fresh fruits and vegetables may be protective. Most cases are idiopathic.

3.26 How does pancreatic cancer present?

The classic presentation is of painless obstructive jaundice (especially in head of pancreas tumours, approximately 60–70%). Patients may also present with abdominal pain with or without weight loss (body, 5–10% and tail, 10–15%, tumours). Pain radiating to the back may be an ominous sign of advanced disease as it implies coeliac plexus involvement and hence the presence of surgically unresectable disease.

3.27 How is pancreatic cancer diagnosed?

Blood tests suggest biliary obstruction and the tumour marker CA19-9 (*see* Q 12.6) may be elevated. This is also raised in acute and chronic pancreatitis and other forms of biliary epithelial malignancy (e.g. cholangiocarcinoma).

Radiology may support the diagnosis and guide best treatment. Ultrasound scanning will reveal a dilated common bile duct and may demonstrate a pancreatic mass as well as liver and lymph node secondaries. CT assesses potential resectability, especially with reference to tumour size, involvement of major vessels and the presence of metastases. CT-guided biopsy may be necessary to confirm the diagnosis if surgical cure is not being contemplated, especially if histology would guide chemotherapy, either clinically or in the setting of a clinical trial of such agents.

3.28 What treatments are available for pancreatic cancer?

Surgical resection is the only chance of long-term cure but unfortunately such surgery is a major undertaking (Whipple's procedure – pancreaticoduodenectomy) with an associated mortality rate of 5% and in any case is only possible in less than 20% of patients with this condition. Even after apparently curative surgery, 5-year survival is only 10–20%, with a median survival of 10–20 months.

Palliative single-agent chemotherapy with gemcitabine is relatively non-toxic and may lead to a slight improvement in quality of life with a modest benefit in terms of longevity (5.7 versus 4.4 months, 18% alive at 12 months, none alive at 18 months).

The mainstay of treatment is often palliative relief of biliary obstruction (either endoscopically or percutaneously with stenting) and pain control.

3.29 What is the prognosis of pancreatic cancer?

Ninety per cent of patients are dead within 1 year of diagnosis. Only 4% are alive after 5 years

 PATIENT QUESTIONS

3.30 The pain I suffer when I get a bout of biliary colic is terrible. My GP says that some painkillers could be harmful – what is the best way to manage the pain?

Simple analgesics (such as paracetamol) are safest and may be effective. Non-steroidal anti-inflammatories such as ibuprofen may also be effective. Stronger analgesics such as opiate drugs (e.g. pethidine, morphine) are often needed. There is no evidence that these drugs make the problem worse.

3.31 What foods should I avoid if I've got gallstones?

It is traditional to recommend a low fat diet, and although there is little hard evidence that this is effective, some patients do find this helpful in reducing both the frequency and severity of attacks of pain.

3.32 Is there much variation in the results of laparoscopic cholecystectomy between different surgeons? Wouldn't I be better off going to a specialist centre rather than to my local hospital?

Laparoscopic cholecystectomy is a now a commonly performed operation with good results achieved by most surgeons. You should discuss different alternatives with your GP.

Jaundice and liver disease

4

4.1 What is jaundice?

Jaundice refers to yellow discolouration of the skin and sclera and is not clinically detectable until the serum bilirubin is greater than 50 μmol/L. Classification of conditions into prehepatic, hepatocellular and posthepatic (cholestatic) is useful but test results may overlap and produce a confusing picture.

Prehepatic jaundice

'Prehepatic' conditions occur 'before' the liver, and as such do not cause any alterations in liver enzymes – alanine transaminase (ALT), aspartate transaminase (AST) and alkaline phosphatase (ALP). These conditions cause an increase in bilirubin levels as a result of:

- increased turnover or destruction of red blood cells (the protoporphyrin ring is broken down into bilirubin), such as autoimmune haemolysis
- reduced processing by the liver (glucuronylation) of bilirubin, such as in neonatal jaundice where the glucuronyl transferase enzyme (which conjugates bilirubin and makes it water soluble) is immature
- Gilbert's syndrome, where the affected person has only half the normal complement of glucuronyl transferase (*see also Q 4.5*).

Hepatocellular jaundice

Hepatocellular jaundice refers to conditions affecting the liver parenchyma (e.g. viral hepatitis), where the insult is directed at the liver cell.

Posthepatic jaundice

Posthepatic jaundice is caused by obstruction to the flow of bile, either within the liver (e.g. primary biliary cirrhosis, primary sclerosing cholangitis) or in the extrahepatic biliary tree (e.g. common bile duct stones, pancreatic carcinoma). A clear and thorough history is essential and will help differentiate between causes.

4.2 What are the common causes of jaundice?

Causes of jaundice – common, uncommon and rare – are outlined in *Table 4.1*.

'Cirrhosis' from any cause (e.g. alcohol, viral, autoimmune) will often give a 'mixed picture' of enzyme abnormality with both hepatic (due to ongoing inflammation) and posthepatic (destruction/compression of bile canaliculi or intrahepatic ducts) components. In established or advanced cirrhosis, the transaminases and alkaline phosphatase levels may be normal or only minimally elevated; the key features to note in this situation are the albumin level and the prothrombin time (PT) or international normalised ratio (INR) which are markers of liver synthetic function.

TABLE 4.1	Causes of jaundice		
	Prehepatic	**Hepatocellular**	**Posthepatic**
Common	Neonatal	Alcohol	Gallstone disease
	Gilbert's syndrome	Drug-induced	Pancreatic carcinoma
		Viral hepatitis	Primary and secondary cancers
Uncommon	Haemolysis	Autoimmune hepatitis	Cholangiocarcinoma
			Sclerosing cholangitis
		Cardiac failure	Pancreatitis
		Pregnancy	Benign strictures
		Haemochromatosis	Lymph node obstruction
			Primary biliary cirrhosis
Rare	Crigler–Najjar	Lymphoma	Parenteral nutrition
		Leptospirosis	Drug-induced
		Alpha-1 antitrypsin deficiency	
		Budd–Chiari syndrome	
		Wilson's disease	

4.3 What is cirrhosis?

Cirrhosis is the final common end result of sustained insult to the liver
from many different causes. It is characterised histologically by fibrosis,
nodular regeneration and architectural disturbance. This process may result
in impeded blood flow through the liver causing portal hypertension and,
when a critical mass of hepatocytes is destroyed, will result in the failure of
the liver's synthetic function. Portal hypertension and hypoalbuminaemia
will eventually lead to ascites.

4.4 What do liver function tests tell us and how do you interpret them?

Liver function tests (LFTs) serve as a guide for further clinical
evaluation of the patient. Different patterns of liver test
abnormalities are useful in narrowing down the potential diagnosis,
and directing further tests. It is important to realise that these
enzymes do not say anything about how well the liver is
'functioning', i.e. maintaining homeostasis. The best markers of liver
function are those that reflect its synthetic ability (albumin and
PT/INR).

Biochemical 'liver tests' are enzymes produced in the liver. ALT and AST – also known as aminotransferases – are produced by the liver cells and are released when damage occurs to the hepatocytes. ALT is relatively specific for the liver, with AST also found in skeletal and cardiac muscle.

Hepatic alkaline phosphatase is synthesised by hepatocytes and in the bile canaliculi. Elevations of hepatic alkaline phosphatase usually indicate blockage to the flow of bile (intra- or extrahepatic).

4.5 What does an isolated hyperbilirubinaemia mean?

An isolated rise in the bilirubin (usually 25–50, though occasionally higher) is usually due to Gilbert's syndrome. This entirely benign jaundice, affecting 4% of the population, is caused by having only half of the glucuronyl transferase activity. As a result, there is a 'back-up' of bilirubin waiting to be conjugated, resulting in a predominantly unconjugated (or 'indirect') hyperbilirubinaemia. Fasting and intercurrent infections increase bilirubin levels in this condition, and the patient may have noticed mild jaundice during previous illnesses.

The important (but rarer) differential diagnosis of an isolated elevated bilirubin is haemolysis. Haemolysis also causes a predominantly unconjugated hyperbilirubinaemia. Measurement of haemoglobin, haptoglobins and reticulocyte count differentiate these two conditions. Haemolysis produces anaemia and releases free haemoglobin into plasma which is 'mopped up' by haptoglobins, thus resulting in decreased levels of haptoglobin. There is also release of new blood cells from the bone marrow to compensate for the destruction of red cells, resulting in a reticulocytosis.

Gilbert's syndrome, once confirmed by the presence of a persisting, mildly raised unconjugated hyperbilirubinaemia, needs no further investigation or follow-up. The most important corollary is that the patient knows the diagnosis, thus preventing further (fruitless) and unnecessary investigations.

4.6 How useful is it for a practice to keep urine dip-stix to test for urobilinogen and bilirubin?

The presence of conjugated bilirubin and the absence of urobilinogen in the urine indicate an obstructive problem, whereas the presence of excess urobilinogen indicates haemolysis. However, the use of urine dip-stix testing has been largely superseded by serum biochemistry and imaging modalities.

4.7 What do raised transaminases (aminotransferases) mean?

Raised transaminases (ALT, AST) are the markers for hepatocellular liver damage.

Moderately raised levels (<500) are non-specific and may be caused by almost any liver disease – for example, viral hepatitis, drug-induced hepatitis, fatty liver (steatosis, non-alcoholic steatohepatitis [NASH], autoimmune liver disease, alcoholic liver disease, etc.).

Markedly elevated levels (>2000) are almost always the result of drug/toxic damage to the liver (e.g. paracetamol overdose), acute viral injury (e.g. hepatitis A, B) or ischaemic injury (e.g. in the context of serious illness, myocardial infarction, sepsis, severe trauma). Occasionally a common bile duct stone may cause a marked rise in the transaminases, but this is usually followed by a rapid drop and subsequent rise in ALP and bilirubin levels.

The ratio of AST:ALT can be useful diagnostically. Most acute liver injury results in an AST:ALT ratio of ≤1. Alcoholic hepatitis, however, characteristically causes an AST:ALT ratio >2, with greater ratios being even more specific for an alcohol aetiology (Cohen & Kaplan 1979).

4.8 What tests are indicated if aminotransferases are elevated?

If the AST/ALT levels are only minimally raised (less than twice normal), it is wise to enquire about alcohol and review medication for possible drug side-effects. If either of these seems likely, abstention or cessation of medication with repeat LFTs after 3 months would be sensible to see if either is responsible.

If the AST/ALT remains elevated, or AST/ALT levels are >2, a simple blood parenchymal liver screen should be undertaken:

- Hepatitis B and C serology
- Autoimmune profile: anti-nuclear antibodies (ANA), anti-smooth muscle antibodies (ASMA), anti-mitochondrial antibodies (AMA)
- Immunoglobulins (IgG raised in autoimmune hepatitis; IgM raised in primary biliary cirrhosis)
- Ferritin (levels >1000 are highly suggestive of haemochromatosis)
- Alpha-1 antitrypsin
- Copper/caeruloplasmin (only indicated in those aged <45).

It is also usual to perform an abdominal ultrasound as a prelude to possible liver biopsy. This may suggest cirrhosis (irregular liver, enlarged spleen) and can exclude a space-occupying lesion within the liver (e.g. metastases), although this usually presents with raised alkaline phosphatase.

Causes of chronically elevated aminotransferases are outlined in *Box 4.1.*

BOX 4.1 Causes of chronically elevated aminotransferases

■ Hepatic causes
   — Non-alcoholic steatosis/steatohepatitis
   — Drug-induced hepatitis
   — Alcohol abuse
   — Autoimmune hepatitis
   — Haemochromatosis/Wilson's disease
   — Alpha-1 antitrypsin deficiency
■ Non-hepatic causes
   — Coeliac disease
   — Inherited disorders of muscle metabolism
   — Acquired muscle diseases
   — Strenuous exercise

Data from Pratt & Kaplan (2000).

4.9 What causes raised alkaline phosphatase?

Alkaline phosphatase (ALP) is produced by the liver, bone, intestine, kidney and placenta. In practice, the important first step is to differentiate between liver and bony ALP, and this is most easily done by checking gamma glutamyl transferase (GGT), which parallels any rise in hepatic alkaline phosphatase.

ALP isoenzymes may also be used to differentiate between liver and bony ALP, but these are more expensive and not always available.

An isolated or predominantly raised hepatic ALP suggests intra- or extrahepatic bile duct obstruction or an infiltrative process such as lymphoma, amyloid, tuberculosis and sarcoidosis.

■ Intrahepatic bile duct obstructive causes include primary and secondary carcinomas, primary sclerosing cholangitis (PSC) and primary biliary cirrhosis (PBC).
■ Extrahepatic bile duct obstructive causes include pancreatic carcinoma, cholangiocarcinoma, common bile duct stones and PSC.

An abdominal ultrasound is *mandatory* if a raised hepatic ALP is the predominant abnormality in order to exclude space-occupying lesions in the liver and pancreas. If dilated intra- and extrahepatic ducts are seen, endoscopic retrograde cholangiopancreatography (ERCP; *see* Q 13.8) or magnetic resonance cholangiopancreatography (MRCP; *see* Q 13.9) is usually indicated.

4.10 What does a raised gamma glutamyl transferase mean?

A raised GGT may be regarded as a 'sensitive form of ALP', or may be inducible by certain drugs.

Elevations of hepatic ALP are always paralleled by rises in GGT. An isolated raised GGT may therefore be a prelude to a raised ALP. Thus, a raised GGT may (rarely) reflect a space-occupying lesion in the liver, although there are often other clinical features which suggest underlying disease in the patient.

It is commonly thought that a raised GGT is suspicious for excess alcohol ingestion; however, other conditions (see Q 4.9) and drugs may also cause raised levels. Alcohol, barbiturates, anti-epileptics and warfarin are all common causes of an inducible raised GGT.

A raised mean cell volume (MCV) in conjunction with a raised GGT is highly suspicious of chronic alcohol excess.

4.11 Should I investigate an isolated raised gamma glutamyl transferase?

Probably not. Many laboratories do not routinely measure GGT when LFTs are requested. It may be worth repeating the LFTs at an interval to make sure that other abnormalities are not developing.

4.12 What is 'fatty liver'/non-alcoholic fatty liver disease?

Non-alcoholic fatty liver disease (NAFLD) comprises the two related conditions of non-alcoholic steatohepatitis (NASH) and steatosis. Histologically, it is virtually identical to alcoholic liver disease, but occurs in the absence of significant alcohol ingestion. It is an extremely common condition, with fatty liver often being noted incidentally on abdominal ultrasound examination.

Its cause is unknown, but there is a strong association with obesity, hyperlipidaemia, diabetes and the metabolic syndrome, and its prevalence mirrors the prevalence of these conditions. It is also associated with certain drugs (e.g. amiodarone, diltiazem, tamoxifen, steroids and anti-retroviral therapy) and with rapid weight loss (e.g. severe starvation, jejunoileal bypass).

The prevalence of fatty liver (on ultrasound) is approximately 10–15% in normal-weight individuals and 70–80% in obese individuals. The prevalence of steatohepatitis (on liver biopsy) is approximately 3% in normal-weight individuals and 15–20% in obese individuals.

4.13 How is non-alcoholic fatty liver disease diagnosed?

NAFLD is often diagnosed after the incidental finding of raised transaminases on biochemical testing. The diagnosis of NAFLD depends on the exclusion of other diseases causing abnormal LFTs (i.e. a negative parenchymal liver screen; *see Q 4.8*). Abdominal ultrasound will often suggest a fatty liver, but is unable to reliably assess the presence of inflammation, fibrosis or cirrhosis.

Whether or not a liver biopsy should be performed is contentious. Histology allows a definitive diagnosis, and also shows whether there is simple steatosis (which appears to have a benign prognosis) or steatohepatitis (with potential to progress to fibrosis and cirrhosis).

4.14 How is non-alcoholic fatty liver disease treated?

Currently this is based on identifying and modifying/treating the factors commonly associated with this condition, namely obesity, hyperlipidaemia and hyperglycaemia. Thus all patients with the diagnosis should have fasting lipids and sugar measured, and treated if necessary. Controlled weight loss should be encouraged in those with a high body mass index, and alcohol and any potentially toxic medications should be discontinued. The role of drug therapy, such as with metformin and statins, is currently being evaluated.

4.15 What is the prognosis in non-alcoholic fatty liver disease?

Good epidemiological data and prospective follow-up data on the natural history of NAFLD are lacking, but NASH would appear to progress to fibrosis in a third and to cirrhosis in up to 20% (Bacon et al 1994, Matteoni et al 1999). Patients therefore need clinical follow-up with serial LFTs approximately every 6 months (specific medication is still an area for future research). The natural history of steatosis is less well understood but is probably benign.

4.16 I have a patient with hyperlipidaemia whom I want to start on a statin. Baseline bloods show mildly raised liver enzymes (AST and ALT) at twice the upper limit of normal. Is it safe to prescribe a statin?

It is a natural instinct amongst physicians to avoid prescribing potentially hepatotoxic drugs to patients with either pre-existing liver disease or abnormal liver enzymes. The *British National Formulary* (BNF) cautions about use of statins in patients with a history of liver disease, and states that treatment should be discontinued if serum transaminase concentration rises to, and persists at, three times the upper limit of the reference range. It also states that statins are contraindicated in active liver disease (or persistently abnormal LFTs).

So what does one do with this sort of scenario? Hyperlipidaemia is associated with NAFLD and therefore substantial numbers of these patients will, in fact, have mildly abnormal transaminases, and yet these are the very patients in whom attention to the management of their hyperlipidaemia (at least from the liver specialist's standpoint) is recommended.

A recent retrospective study has addressed this issue. In the report, three cohorts of patients were followed:

■ cohort 1 were hyperlipidaemic patients with elevated baseline transaminases ([mean ± SD] ALT 43 ± 23 IU/L; AST 55 ± 37) who were prescribed a statin
■ cohort 2 were hyperlipidaemic patients with normal transaminases who were prescribed a statin
■ cohort 3 were patients with elevated liver enzymes ([mean ± SD] ALT 61 ± 47 IU/L; AST 57 ± 49) who were not prescribed a statin.

All cohorts excluded patients abusing alcohol or with evidence of hepatitis B and/or C infection (therefore presumably consisting mostly of patients with NAFLD). Elevations in liver enzymes in the 6-month follow-up period were categorised as 'mild–moderate' if AST and/or ALT rose up to 10-fold above the upper limit of normal (or above baseline in those with pre-existing elevations); 'severe' elevations were categorised as the development of serum bilirubin >3 mg/dl (regardless of baseline transaminases) or elevations of transaminases greater than 10-fold from their starting point.

Although cohort 1 had a higher incidence of mild–moderate liver enzyme elevations compared to cohort 2 – 4.7% versus 1.9%, respectively (p = 0.002) – there was no significant difference in the frequency of severe elevations – 0.6% versus 0.2%, respectively (p = 0.2). More enlightening, however, was the finding that there was no difference in mild–moderate elevations between cohort 1 and cohort 3 – 4.7% versus 6.4%, respectively (p = 0.2) – or in severe elevations – 0.6% versus 0.4%, respectively (p = 0.6). This suggests that the elevations seen in cohort 1 were due to the intrinsic liver disease itself, rather than as a result of the prescribed statin (Chalasani et al 2004).

It would therefore seem reasonable to treat hyperlipidaemic patients with mildly raised transaminases (up to three times the upper limit of normal) with a statin if desired. LFTs should be checked after 1–3 months, and then 6-monthly for a year (as per the BNF guidelines), and the statin stopped only if the liver enzymes exceed three times the upper limit of normal.

HEPATITIS A

4.17 What is hepatitis A?

This is the commonest viral hepatitis. It is a benign, self-limiting infection with no chronicity. It is spread by the faecal–oral route and is most common in areas of poor sanitation and poor quality water supply. As well as person-to-person contact, it may also be acquired from eating raw or undercooked shellfish, which filter sewage.

4.18 How is hepatitis A diagnosed?

In infants and children the condition is often subclinical and not diagnosed. This is typical in areas of high prevalence such as Africa, Asia, and Central and South America. In Northern and Western Europe, North America, Canada and Australia, peak infection rates occur in adolescents and young adults.

Typically, there is a prodrome of lethargy and general malaise, anorexia, nausea and vomiting. ALT levels are often >500 units per litre. Jaundice (approximately 30% of adults and <5% children) and pruritus may develop. Detection of IgM anti-hepatitis A virus confirms the diagnosis.

4.19 How is hepatitis A treated?

There is no specific treatment. Hospitalisation is only recommended in those with severe anorexia or vomiting, or those developing acute liver failure. Colestyramine may be used for pruritus. A short course of prednisolone may be given to those with severe cholestasis.

4.20 What is the prognosis in hepatitis A?

Excellent. Most patients have recovered within 2 months. Infection in children is less severe and has a mortality of 0.1%. Severity of illness and mortality rates increase with age and are approximately 1% for those over 40 years old.

4.21 How can hepatitis A be prevented?

Strict personal hygiene is important in preventing person-to-person spread, especially in hospitals or institutions. Passive immunity (by intramuscular injection of pooled human immunoglobulin) is 85–95% effective in preventing infection in exposed individuals and lasts for 4–6 months. It may also prevent or attenuate infection if it is given within 1–2 weeks of exposure. Live attenuated and inactivated vaccines are highly effective, with a protective efficacy of 95–100%, and have a duration of over 20 years.

HEPATITIS B

4.22 What is hepatitis B?

It is estimated that over 300 million (5%) of the world population are chronically infected with hepatitis B virus (HBV). Acquisition of the virus in adulthood usually results in clearance of the virus, with only about 5% becoming chronically infected (chronic carriers), as defined by persistence of the virus 6 months after initial infection (*Box 4.2*). The risk of chronic infection is much higher in infants.

Transmission may be parenteral or vertical:

BOX 4.2 Hepatitis serology tests

Test	Outcome
All hepatitis serology negative	No history of infection
sAg positive, eAg negative, cAb positive	Carrier – low infectivity risk
sAg positive, eAg positive, cAb positive	Carrier – high infectivity risk
sAg negative (therefore eAg negative), sAb positive, cAb positive	Successfully cleared infection from body
sAb positive, cAb negative	Successful immunisation

'Carriage' or being a 'carrier' of the virus is synonymous with having active infection.
cAb is seen only in those who have been exposed to the natural (wild) virus.
cAb, core antibody; eAg, e antigen; sAb, surface antibody; sAg, surface antigen.

■ Parenteral transmission is via blood/blood products or mucous membranes. Risk factors include blood transfusion, dialysis, 'unsafe' sexual practices, intravenous drug abuse, tattooing, acupuncture and working in a healthcare setting. The virus is detectable in semen and saliva, which represent possible sources of infection.

■ In vertical transmission, 70–90% of babies born to high viral load hepatitis B e-antigen-positive mothers acquire the infection.

4.23 How is hepatitis B diagnosed?

Acute HBV infection may be subclinical or, at the other extreme, present with jaundice. The incubation period is 2–6 months. Hepatitis B surface antigen (HBsAg), which marks active infection, and hepatitis B e-antigen (HBeAg) and HBV DNA – both indicative of active viral replication (and therefore greater potential infectivity) – may be detected approximately 6 weeks after exposure to the virus. ALT/AST levels are usually >500 units per litre. IgM, followed by IgG anti-core antibody (anti-HBc), then develop. Clearance of the virus is associated with falling levels of HBsAg and development of anti-sAb (again IgM and then IgG), the latter indicating immunity to the virus.

4.24 How is hepatitis B treated?

Acute HBV infection does not need any active treatment, as 95% of infected individuals will clear the virus. A rising prothrombin time and/or decreasing albumin, indicating a failing liver, necessitate close hospital monitoring and, if progressive, transfer to a liver transplant centre. In chronic HBV infection, alpha-interferon has been shown to clear the virus in up to one-third of cases (loss of HBV DNA and HBeAg). Trials using oral lamivudine for 1 year have shown similar results.

Patients with high pretreatment aminotransferase levels are most likely to respond to either treatment; those with low pretreatment serum HBV DNA levels, histologically active hepatitis and short duration of infection are most likely to respond to interferon.

> **Follow-up for patients who are carriers of the virus (i.e. have active infection)**
> Patients who acquire hepatitis B at an early age (especially in the neonatal period) are at high risk of developing hepatomas and cirrhosis. These patients should undergo periodic surveillance with alphafetoprotein, LFTs and abdominal ultrasound examination at 4- to 6-monthly intervals (*see also Q 4.52*).
> Patients who acquire hepatitis B at a later age are at less risk of developing hepatoma, but should probably have alphafetoprotein and LFTs measured every 6 months and receive an annual liver ultrasound scan. It is reasonable for this surveillance to occur in primary care. However, if the results of these tests indicate deteriorating liver function, referral to a specialist clinic is recommended; if they show the presence of a hepatoma, urgent referral is mandatory.
>
> **Follow-up for patients who have successfully cleared the virus from their body**
> Nil is required unless they have already developed cirrhosis, in which case periodic surveillance with alphafetoprotein and abdominal ultrasound examination at 4- to 6-monthly intervals would seem appropriate (*see also Q 4.52*).

4.25 What is the prognosis in hepatitis B?

Less than 1% of those with acute HBV infection develop acute liver failure, and overall mortality is 1–3%.

The risk of chronic HBV infection is related to age of acquisition, with neonates of infected mothers having an up to 90% chance of chronic infection compared to <5% if acquired as an adult. Immunocompetency is also important. Coexisting human immunodeficiency virus (HIV) infection confers a 20–30% risk of chronic HBV infection; those on immunosuppressive therapy or chemotherapy for cancer are also at higher risk of chronic disease.

The prognosis of chronic HBV infection is related to the presence of active viral replication, with approximately 20% developing cirrhosis over 5 years. Prognosis is also determined by the underlying degree of liver damage. In a USA study, 5-year survival of chronic HBV-infected patients ranged from 97% in those with minimal inflammation to 55% in those with established cirrhosis (Weissberg et al 1984).

4.26 How can hepatitis B be prevented?

Screening of blood and blood products for HBV and safer sexual practices have reduced incidence in developed countries.

Passive immunisation with hepatitis B immune globulin (HBIG) is effective and is given to neonates of HBV-infected mothers (where it is approximately 90% effective in preventing transmission) and also following needlestick injury or sexual exposure. It should be given as soon as possible following needlestick injury, ideally within the first 48 hours.

Active immunisation is highly effective, inducing an antibody response in over 95% of recipients.

4.27 What is the likely future management of hepatitis B?

Future management will ideally include the development of more efficacious anti-viral agents, including the utilisation of multidrug regimens. The key to the more effective management of hepatitis B infection worldwide is widespread vaccination programmes.

HEPATITIS C

4.28 What is hepatitis C?

Hepatitis C infection is widespread, estimated to affect 3% of the population worldwide. Transmission is parenteral, like hepatitis B. The chief risk factor for its spread in the UK and Western world is intravenous drug abuse. Prior to 1991 blood was not screened for hepatitis C virus (HCV) and so blood transfusions, blood products and haemodialysis were also risk factors for acquisition of the virus.

Unlike HBV, HCV is not usually cleared by the body, and approximately 80–90% of exposed individuals remain chronically infected. Infection is often asymptomatic, or may produce a 'flu-like' illness. It presents acutely with jaundice in less than 10%.

4.29 How is hepatitis C diagnosed?

Anti-HCV antibodies are detected in the blood of exposed individuals, with polymerase chain reaction (PCR) used to confirm the presence of virus.

The transaminase enzymes may be normal or only minimally elevated, and are not reliable indicators of inflammation in the liver. It is for this reason, as well as the absence of other reliable markers of disease progression, that infected individuals should be followed up by a specialist clinic and generally offered a liver biopsy to allow assessment of the degree of inflammation, necrosis and fibrosis of the liver parenchyma.

4.30 How is hepatitis C treated?

Combined treatment with pegylated interferon and oral ribavirin will clear the virus in approximately 50% of infected individuals. It is a costly treatment, may have significant side-effects, and patients often experience general malaise and 'flu-like' symptoms throughout the treatment period (usually 6 months). It is therefore a considerable undertaking.

4.31 What is the prognosis in hepatitis C?

The virus is generally indolent. It takes approximately 20–30 years for cirrhosis to develop. A few individuals show more aggressive disease, with the onset of cirrhosis within 10 years of infection. Excess alcohol is synergistic. As treatment is only successful in one-half of patients, may cause significant morbidity, and the natural history of the condition is relatively benign, those patients with only minimal inflammation on liver biopsies may elect to defer treatment. Hepatitis C virus is oncogenic and, as such, is an additional risk factor for the development of hepatoma, over and above that conferred by the presence of cirrhosis.

4.32 What are the likely future developments in viral hepatitis?

The development of more efficacious anti-viral agents. No vaccine or postexposure prophylaxis is currently available and this provides an opportunity for improved management in the future. Education and counselling remain essential to limit spread of infection.

HAEMOCHROMATOSIS

4.33 What is haemochromatosis?

This is an autosomal recessive condition characterised by the excess accumulation of iron within the body. It is a relatively common condition, affecting approximately 1 in 400 of the population. It is underdiagnosed since it does not usually produce any symptoms or signs until the onset of cirrhosis and decompensated liver disease (ascites or jaundice).

Excess iron is deposited in the liver, exciting an inflammatory response, which over years may result in cirrhosis. Other organs – including the myocardium, pancreas and pituitary – can be affected, often impairing their normal function.

Iron accumulation is slow and lifelong, and many patients do not present until the fifth or sixth decade of life with decompensated liver disease. Women are protected by menstruation, and therefore present at a much later age.

4.34 How is haemochromatosis diagnosed?

Often the diagnosis is not made until the patient presents with advanced liver disease. It may be picked up earlier on the chance finding of abnormal liver function tests for other reasons.

> A raised ferritin (especially if greater than 1000 mcg/l) is suspicious for the disease (see parenchymal liver screen, Q 4.8), although liver inflammation from any cause may release iron and result in elevated ferritin levels (commonly elevated, but rarely above 300 mcg/l).
>   The transferrin saturation (serum iron divided by total iron binding capacity × 100%) is the most sensitive and specific non-genetic blood test for haemochromatosis, with saturations above 45% being abnormal.

It has recently been discovered that over 90% of patients with genetic haemochromatosis have one of two distinct mutations in the HFE gene, which results in haemochromatosis: C282Y, in which tyrosine is substituted for cysteine, and H63D where a histidine is substituted for an aspartate. These mutations may be detected via a blood sample, and represent the HFE gene test.

Liver biopsy is the gold standard for diagnosis, demonstrating an increase in the dry weight of hepatic iron. If clinical suspicion is high, or an individual is found to have a positive HFE gene test in the setting of abnormal LFTs, it is usual practice to obtain a liver biopsy. This allows a definitive diagnosis and also detects the presence or absence of cirrhosis. The HFE gene test should be offered as a screening test to other members of the family of an affected person. In individuals who are found to be homozygous for C282Y, or are compound heterozygotes (C282Y/H63D), a liver biopsy is not necessary if they are young, have normal LFTs and a ferritin <1000. In these individuals, therapeutic phlebotomy should begin to reduce the ferritin to less than 50.

4.35 How is haemochromatosis treated?

Serial venesection is required, until the serum ferritin is in the low/normal range. This may require as many as 30 or 40 weekly venesections. Once achieved, venesection is usually needed only once every 3–6 months.

4.36 What is the prognosis in haemochromatosis?

This is dependent on the stage and severity of liver disease at the time of diagnosis. If the disease is diagnosed and treated before the onset of diabetes or cirrhosis, then prognosis is excellent with no increased mortality compared to the general population. Haemochromatosis imparts an extra risk factor over and above cirrhosis for the development of hepatoma.

4.37 What is the likely future management of haemochromatosis?

This is a relatively common condition affecting approximately 1 in 400 of the population. Genetic testing of offspring of affected individuals ensures early detection and treatment.

AUTOIMMUNE HEPATITIS

4.38 What is autoimmune hepatitis?

Autoimmune hepatitis is an uncommon condition, characterised by an immune response directed against the liver. It is more common in women, and often presents acutely with jaundice. Untreated, mortality is as high as 50% by 3 years.

4.39 How is autoimmune hepatitis diagnosed?

Individuals may present with general malaise, arthralgia, fever and weight loss. LFTs show a transaminitis. Serology most commonly reveals positive anti-smooth muscle antibodies (ASMA) or anti-nuclear antibodies (ANA) (type 1) with a raised serum IgG. Other variants include anti-liver/kidney/microsomal (anti-LKM) antibody-positive individuals (type 2) and those with anti-soluble liver antigen/liver pancreas (anti-SLA/LP) antibodies (type 3). Liver biopsy usually shows characteristic changes.

4.40 How is autoimmune hepatitis treated?

Prednisolone at a dose of 40–60 mg is usually instituted with gradual tapering once the LFTs have normalised. The average duration of treatment to produce remission is 2 years. Relapse is common, with one-half relapsing within 6 months and three-quarters relapsing within 3 years. Azathioprine may be used as a steroid-sparing agent.

4.41 What is the prognosis in autoimmune hepatitis?

Treatment improves prognosis, with 10-year survival rates of approximately 90%.

4.42 What does the future hold for those suffering from autoimmune hepatitis?

Further insight into the pathogenesis of the condition and the development of more efficacious immunosuppressive agents.

ALCOHOLIC LIVER DISEASE

4.43 What is alcoholic liver disease?

This is the commonest cause of cirrhosis in the UK and the Western world. Individual sensitivity to alcohol varies, and the result of excess consumption may range from no insult through to fatty liver (steatosis), steatohepatitis, fibrosis and cirrhosis. A bout of increased or excessive consumption may cause an acute alcoholic hepatitis, a serious condition with significant associated mortality.

4.44 How is alcoholic liver disease diagnosed?

The diagnosis is usually evident on the history. It is still usual to perform a parenchymal liver screen (*see* Q 4.8), since alcoholics are not immune from other liver diseases. Occasionally the drinking history is concealed. Suggestive indicators of alcohol abuse are a raised MCV in conjunction with a raised GGT, and a transaminitis with an AST:ALT ratio >2. A liver biopsy may show characteristic or supportive features and also confirm or rule out the presence of cirrhosis.

4.45 How is alcoholic liver disease treated?

First line treatment is reduction of alcohol consumption to within recommended limits (if no significant liver disease) or abstinence in those with advanced liver disease. Alcoholic hepatitis will often settle with withdrawal of alcohol. A 1-month course of steroids may reduce mortality and there is also evidence for the use of pentoxifylline (an anti-tumour necrosis factor compound).

4.46 What is the prognosis in alcoholic liver disease?

If the patient has established cirrhosis, the 5-year survival is greater than 60% if abstinent, but less than 40% if drinking continues. In alcoholic cirrhotics without complications (varices, ascites), the 5-year survival approaches 90% if they remain abstinent. The worst prognosis group is cirrhotic patients with complications who continue to drink; their median survival is 2 years, with approximately one-third surviving 5 years.

FURTHER MANAGEMENT

4.47 Which patients need a liver biopsy?

Liver biopsy is indicated for (confirming) diagnosis and assessing severity (staging) of disease. In general terms, patients with the following conditions will need biopsies:

■ hepatitis B (chronic)
■ hepatitis C
■ suspected autoimmune hepatitis
■ suspected primary biliary cirrhosis
■ suspected haemochromatosis
■ unexplained transaminitis (significant)
■ suspected alcoholic liver disease.

The patient must understand that liver biopsy in the context of unexplained abnormal LFTs has a 20% chance of altering management (although not necessarily prognosis), but is associated with complications and risk (*see Ch. 13*). However, opinion is still divided about the role of liver biopsy in asymptomatic raised transaminases in the face of negative serological and viral markers.

A study of over 350 such patients (aminotransferases more than double normal for at least 6 months) revealed only 6% to have entirely normal biopsies, with 18% of patients having their management directly altered by the biopsy findings. Fibrosis was found in 20% and cirrhosis in 6%. The commonest finding was 'fatty liver' (Skelly et al 2001).

4.48 Which patients need an ultrasound scan?

Any patient with persistently abnormal LFTs (other than an isolated hyperbilirubinaemia, i.e. Gilbert's syndrome/haemolysis) warrants an ultrasound scan. Essentially this will help decide whether this is a posthepatic (extrahepatic biliary obstruction, e.g. common bile duct stones, carcinoma of the pancreas) or hepatic problem (e.g. NASH, hepatitis C, alcoholic liver disease, etc.) and dictate further investigations.

4.49 Which patients do not need to be seen by a gastroenterologist?

Patients with Gilbert's syndrome, haemolysis (may require haematological referral) or acute self-limiting viral hepatitis (e.g. hepatitis A, cytomegalovirus, Epstein–Barr virus) without systemic upset.

4.50 What is the current treatment and prognosis in liver disease?

Current treatment and prognosis in hepatitis B, hepatitis C, autoimmune hepatitis, primary biliary cirrhosis, haemochromatosis and alcoholic liver disease are outlined in *Table 4.2*.

4.51 What is the difference between a hepatoma and a hepatocellular carcinoma?

Nothing – the terms are synonymous.

TABLE 4.2 Treatment and prognosis in liver disease

Condition	Treatment	Prognosis
Hepatitis B	Interferon with lamivudine in high-risk patients	10–40% progress to cirrhosis over 10 years; 3–6% develop hepatocellular carcinoma per annum[1]
Hepatitis C	Interferon plus ribavirin	3–4% per annum develop hepatocellular carcinoma
Autoimmune hepatitis	Prednisolone plus azathioprine	Depends on degree of inflammation. Those in remission have 90% 10-year life expectancy[2]
Primary biliary cirrhosis	Ursodeoxycholic acid (may not affect mortality and recent meta-analysis does not recommend its use)[3]	Asymptomatic: mean survival 16 years; symptomatic: mean survival 8 years
		Liver transplant curative
Alcoholic liver disease	Steroids of use in severe alcoholic hepatitis	If decompensated (ascites), approximately 50% 2-year survival

[1] Di Marco et al (1999); [2] Roberts et al (1996); [3] Goulis et al (1999).

4.52 Who is at risk of developing hepatocellular carcinoma?

Certain groups are at increased risk of developing HCC (hepatocellular carcinoma, hepatoma), i.e. those with:

- cirrhosis of any cause (3–4% per annum)
- haemochromatosis*
- hepatitis B- and C-induced cirrhosis.*

The value of screening for the development of HCC in these conditions is controversial. Some adopt a policy of serum alphafetoprotein and ultrasound every 6 months.

(* These conditions are at particularly increased risk.)

PATIENT QUESTIONS

4.53 What medications should I avoid (and for how long), and when can I drink alcohol again after an attack of viral hepatitis?

Hepatotoxic drugs and abstinence from alcohol is usually recommended for 3–6 months after the onset of symptoms. Paracetamol is probably safe throughout the illness; however, most physicians recommend it is avoided while jaundice persists.

4.54 I have had viral hepatitis previously. What is the risk of passing the virus on to my partner or children?

The risk depends on the type of virus you had (A, B or C), and whether you still have the virus (i.e. carrier status).

■ *Hepatitis A*: The risk of spread in acute infection is chiefly via the faecal–oral route. Theoretically it could be transmitted via sharing of needles in the acute viraemic phase. There is no carrier state, and therefore no risk of spread once the acute illness is over.

■ *Hepatitis B*: Most patients clear the virus and pose no risk of infecting others. A small minority (5%) become carriers of the virus. Infection may be spread by blood (sharing needles) or unprotected sex, especially if the carrier is of high infectivity ('e' antigen positive). Partners of chronic carriers should all be offered vaccination.

Vertical transmission (i.e. from mother to baby during birth) depends on carrier status. If the mother is of relatively low infectivity (surface antigen positive only), the risk of transmission to the baby is 10–40%. However, if the mother is of high infectivity (e-antigen positive), the risk is as high as 90%.

■ *Hepatitis C*: In contrast to hepatitis B, most patients infected with hepatitis C become chronic carriers and may potentially transmit the virus via blood or unprotected sex. The risk of both sexual and vertical transmission is low, being less than 5% and between 0 and 10%, respectively.

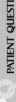

Iron deficiency anaemia

5

5.1   How is iron deficiency anaemia (IDA) defined?

The World Health Organization defines anaemia as a haemoglobin (Hb) of less than 13 g/dl for a man and less than 12g/dl for a woman. It is best, however, to use the local laboratory range as this aims to reflect the normal range for the population in that region.

A low mean corpuscular volume (MCV) is suggestive of iron deficiency, but beta-thalassaemia trait, as well as sickle cell trait, result in a mild anaemia with a characteristically very low MCV. The likelihood ratio (LR) of an MCV >74 but ≤85 actually reflecting true iron deficiency is only 1.35, but at lower levels (MCV <74) the LR rises to 8.82, i.e. a patient with an MCV of 72 is almost ninefold more likely to be iron deficient than a patient with an MCV >85. The best measure of iron deficiency is by bone marrow examination, and this is occasionally required; however, in practical terms, the best marker is serum ferritin. A serum ferritin <18 mcg/l gives a LR of 41.4 of that person actually being iron deficient.

5.2   What does a positive likelihood ratio mean?

A likelihood [positive] ratio is defined as the sensitivity of the test divided by 1 – specificity. If a test has a sensitivity of 90% and a specificity of 90%, then the likelihood of a positive test actually reflecting the truth is 0.9/0.1 = 9, i.e. the patient with the positive test is nine times more likely to have the condition being tested for than a patient who has negative result. In clinical practice, a LR >10 is considered useful.

5.3   How common is iron deficiency anaemia?

Iron deficiency anaemia is the most common of all the anaemias in all countries. Its prevalence is 2–5% in adult men and postmenopausal women, and it affects 5–10% of menstruating women.

5.4   How much iron does the body need each day?

Total body iron is 2000–3000 mg for women and 2500–4000 mg for men. Two-thirds is contained in circulating haemoglobin, with most of the remainder being stored as ferritin and haemosiderin in the reticuloendothelial system. A small percentage of ferritin is present in the serum, and its level correlates with iron stores in the reticuloendothelial system.

Every day the body loses 0.5–1 mg of iron in the urine, sweat and faeces. This is normally balanced by the equivalent absorption of iron from the gastrointestinal tract. The average Western diet contains about 10–15 mg of iron per day. Iron is relatively poorly absorbed. The normal person absorbs between 5 and 10% of the dietary iron (i.e. 0.5–1 mg per day) and this can only be increased two- to threefold in states of increased requirement (e.g. pregnancy) or deficiency. Thus, loss or utilisation of more than 2.5 mg iron per day results in iron depletion. There is approximately 0.5 mg of iron in 1 ml of blood. It can therefore be seen that chronic blood loss of as little as 5 ml daily will deplete the iron stores and eventually result in iron deficiency anaemia.

5.5 How much iron is contained in common iron preparations?

Ferrous sulphate is the most commonly prescribed preparation. Each 200 mg tablet contains 67 mg of iron. Ferrous gluconate contains 37 mg of iron in each 300 mg tablet.

5.6 What is ferritin?

Ferritin is a water-soluble complex of iron and protein. Most is stored in the reticuloendothelial system. Serum ferritin, which reflects the iron stores, is the best marker of iron deficiency outside of a bone marrow examination. It is, however, an acute phase protein and levels may be falsely elevated in inflammatory states. Levels are also very high in acute hepatitis. Serum iron and total iron binding capacity (TIBC) are less powerful tests for measuring iron deficiency.

5.7 What is transferrin?

The majority of iron is transported in the circulation bound to transferrin, an iron-binding protein. This protein delivers iron to the bone marrow where it is utilised in developing red blood cells and also to the spleen and liver (reticuloendothelial system) for storage.

5.8 What is transferrin saturation?

This is the percentage of transferrin that is bound to iron. It is calculated by dividing the iron concentration by the total iron binding capacity × 100%. It is the most sensitive indicator of pathological iron overload. Patients with haemochromatosis (*see Q 4.34*) have transferrin saturations >60% (males) and >45% (females).

5.9 What are the causes of iron deficiency anaemia?

Iron deficiency may be caused by inadequate intake (<5%), poor absorption (<5%) or excessive loss (90%). Menstruation results in an average loss of about 70 ml of blood per month and thus places a large demand on the available iron stores in the body.

Occult blood loss may occur from the urinary system (either dip-stix testing or laboratory microscopy of a midstream urine sample should always be performed in every patient who presents with IDA) but the most common route is the gastrointestinal tract.

5.10 What abnormalities in the gastrointestinal tract may cause iron deficiency anaemia?

There are many lesions capable of causing IDA, including:

- erosive oesophagitis and gastritis
- peptic ulcers
- gastric polyps and carcinoma
- multiple vascular ectasias (e.g. angiodysplasia)
- coeliac disease
- inflammatory bowel disease
- colonic polyps
- colorectal carcinoma (CRC).

> Iron deficiency anaemia should never be attributed to the presence of a hiatus hernia or diverticulosis.
>
> Diverticular disease and oesophageal varices are not regarded as causing chronic iron deficiency anaemia, since they are associated with causing acute bleeds – frank per rectum bleeds or haematemesis, respectively.

5.11 Do aspirin and non-steroidal anti-inflammatory drugs (NSAIDs) cause iron deficiency anaemia?

Although aspirin and NSAIDs may cause oesophagitis, gastritis, peptic ulcers and small intestinal ulceration – and therefore result in gastrointestinal bleeding – there are no data showing that patients on aspirin, for example, are more likely to suffer from iron deficiency anaemia. Indeed, patients on low dose aspirin have been found to have only minimally (and therefore unlikely to be significant) increased faecal blood, and low dose aspirin or warfarin alone does not appear to cause a positive faecal occult blood test (FOBT).

5.12 Should all people with iron deficiency anaemia be investigated/referred for investigation?

> There have been relatively few prospective studies on the investigation of iron deficiency anaemia (*Table 5.1*), but most would advocate examination of both the upper and lower gastrointestinal tract.
>
> The British Society of Gastroenterology (BSG) guidelines (Goddard et al 2000) suggest that all men and postmenopausal women who are found to have IDA should be investigated with both upper and

lower gastrointestinal tract evaluation, since important dual pathology occurs in around 5% of cases (*Fig. 5.1*).

In the published studies, several of the colorectal carcinomas discovered have been associated with oesophagitis or peptic ulcer disease. Overall, approximately 10% of men and postmenopausal women will harbour a colorectal cancer, 5% gastric carcinoma, and up to 5% will have coeliac disease. No cause will be found in approximately 25% of all patients investigated.

5.13 Do premenopausal women need investigation or can the anaemia be attributed to menstruation?

There are several published studies on the investigation of iron deficiency anaemia in premenopausal women (*Table 5.2*).

In the largest study, the upper and lower gastrointestinal tracts of 186 premenopausal women were examined prospectively by gastroscopy, duodenal biopsies and colonoscopy. Pathology was found in 13%. None of the 175 who had duodenal biopsies had coeliac disease. Five (3%) gastric and six (3%) colorectal carcinomas were discovered. All cases were aged 41 years or over, and 8/11 had abdominal symptoms or were faecal occult blood positive. Predictors of malignancy were Hb <10, faecal occult blood positivity, abdominal symptoms or greater than 5 kg weight loss.

In a smaller study, colonic carcinoma was discovered in 3/111 (2.7%) premenopausal women, and all (including four discovered to have inflammatory bowel disease and one with a colonic ulcer) were positive on faecal occult blood testing (Green & Rockey 2004).

A further national prospective cohort study found no diagnosed cases of gastrointestinal malignancy in 442 premenopausal women with iron deficiency (92 with anaemia, 350 without) during a 2-year follow-up period (Iannou et al 2003).

Most menstruating females have a physiological explanation for their IDA. The BSG recommends that, in the absence of gastrointestinal symptoms, premenopausal women under the age of 50 should have an anti-endomysial antibody test to exclude coeliac disease. Only patients with upper gastrointestinal symptoms should have gastroscopy and duodenal biopsies. Colonoscopy under the age of 50 should only be performed if there are colonic symptoms, a strong family history of CRC (one first degree relative <45 years, or two first degree relatives of any age) or persistent iron deficiency anaemia following iron repletion and correction of any underlying cause (e.g. menorrhagia, blood donation).

TABLE 5.1 Prospective studies of the investigation of iron deficiency anaemia

Author	N	Upper (%)	Lower (%)	Dual (%)	Coeliac (%)	no△ (%)	UCA (%)	LCA (%)
Kerlin et al (1979)	100	74	22	n/a	[2]	3	6	12
Cook et al (1986)	100	60	23	7	0	14	6	14
Rockey & Cello (1993)	100	37	26	1	noD2	38	1	11
McIntyre & Long (1993)	111	41	16	2	6	34	7	5
Kepczyk & Kadakia (1995)	70	56	30	17	6	29	6	5
Bampton & Holloway (1996)	80	48	20	7	1	40	1	9
Hardwick & Armstrong (1997)*	89	57	56	29	[2]	10	10	37

Coeliac, percentage identified to have coeliac disease ([ ] indicates that not all patients in these studies had duodenal biopsies, therefore the values may be underestimates); Dual, percentage in whom there was important upper and lower gastrointestinal tract pathology; Lower, yield of lower gastrointestinal tract investigation; N, number in trial; n/a, not applicable; no△, no diagnosis found after upper and lower gastrointestinal tract evaluation; noD2, no duodenal biopsies were taken; UCA/LCA, percentage of upper (UCA) and lower (LCA) gastrointestinal tract cancers identified; Upper, yield of upper gastrointestinal tract investigation.

* This publication has a disproportionately high number of colorectal carcinomas. It is noteworthy that this was a surgical practice and presumably the high percentage of colorectal carcinomas was a reflection of the pattern of referral to this service.

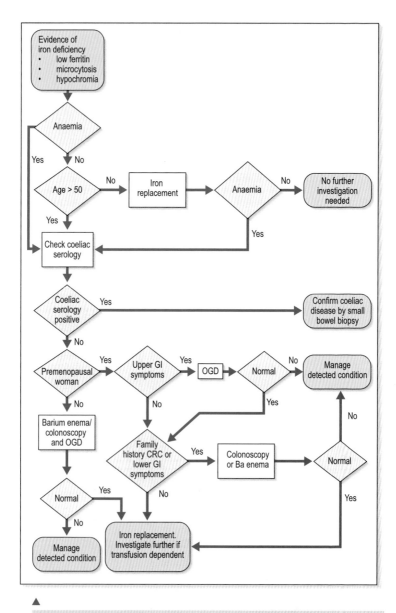

▲

Fig. 5.1 Management of iron deficiency in adults. Ba enema, barium enema; CRC, colorectal cancer; OGD, gastroscopy. (Reproduced with permission from the British Society of Gastroenterology.)

TABLE 5.2 Prospective studies of the investigation of iron deficiency anaemia in premenopausal women

Author	N	Upper (%)	Lower (%)	Dual (%)	Coeliac (%)	noΔ (%)	UCA (%)	LCA (%)
Bini et al (1998)	186	7	6	0	[0]	87	3	3
Kepczyk et al (1999)	19	95	5	5	n/a	5	0	0

See Table 5.1 for key to abbreviations.

TABLE 5.3 Prospective studies of the investigation of iron deficiency alone

Author	N	Upper (%)	Lower (%)	UCA (%)	LCA (%)
Joosten et al (1993)*	13 Fe	38	8	0	8
	15 IDA	40	13	7	13
Lee et al (1998)†	143	40	23	1	9
	(43% Fe)				
Joosten et al (1999)*	55 Fe	56	16	5	9
	96 IDA	49	32	2	14

Fe, iron deficiency only (no anaemia); IDA, iron deficiency anaemia; Lower, pathology yield from colonoscopy; N, number of patients in study; UCA/LCA, percentage of upper (UCA) and lower (LCA) gastrointestinal tract cancers identified; Upper, pathology yield from gastroscopy.

* All patients in these studies were elderly inpatients (mean age 83 years) screened for iron deficiency on admission.
† No significant difference in findings between those patients with Hb above and below 13 g/dl, i.e. between those with IDA and isolated iron deficiency.

5.14 Should isolated iron deficiency without anaemia be investigated?

It is unusual to be confronted with such scenarios, since serum ferritin is usually measured after the anaemia is discovered.

As iron deficiency predates the development of anaemia, it would seem reasonable to apply the same rules as for those who are actually anaemic. There is, however, very little published on this subject (*Table 5.3*).

It would seem that approximately 10% of those with iron deficiency alone are found to have a colorectal carcinoma, supporting the idea that this group of patients should be investigated in the same way as those who are actually anaemic.

The most recent BSG guidelines (Goddard et al 2000) on the investigation of iron deficiency anaemia suggest that patients over the age of 50 (men and women) who have isolated iron deficiency should have their upper and lower gastrointestinal tract investigated (*see Fig. 5.1*).

5.15 For how long should patients be treated with iron?

Oral iron therapy should be given to correct the anaemia (the haemoglobin will rise at approximately 1 g/dl every 7–10 days), and then for a further 3 months to replenish the iron stores.

5.16 How long should I follow up people who have been investigated for IDA?

The BSG recommends that a full blood count is performed at 3-monthly intervals for 1 year following normalisation of anaemia, and a single further check 1 year later.

5.17 What should be done for those patients in whom no cause for the anaemia is found?

These patients should similarly have their blood counts checked at 3-monthly intervals for 1 year and again 1 year later. It does not appear that sinister pathology is missed in this group. A retrospective questionnaire study from Lincoln looked at 93 patients with no cause found for their anaemia following gastroscopy and barium enema. Questionnaires were returned from general practitioners for 89 out of the 93 patients: 6 patients had relocated, leaving 83 patients with a mean follow-up of 6.1 years (range 4–12 years). Of these, 10 patients had died, all of non-gastrointestinal causes; 15 were still on iron and all had a normal haemoglobin level; 58 were not on iron, with 8 having a mild anaemia (Hb 11.2–13.4 g/dl) (Sahay & Scott 1993).

5.18 What should I do if the iron deficiency anaemia recurs?

If iron deficiency anaemia recurs after evaluation of the upper and lower gastrointestinal tract, oral iron should be re-prescribed. If this fails to normalise and maintain the haemoglobin, further investigation may be necessary. In such cases, it would seem sensible to perform a colonoscopy if initial lower gastrointestinal tract examination was performed by means of a barium enema, since colonoscopy has greater accuracy and may detect angiodysplasia which cannot be picked up radiologically.

If the iron deficiency anaemia becomes transfusion dependent, small bowel meal, small bowel enteroscopy and video capsule endoscopy (*see Ch. 13*) should be considered. Mesenteric angiography may demonstrate vascular malformations, and diagnostic laparotomy with on-table small bowel enteroscopy may be useful in difficult cases.

Small bowel radiology has very low yield in the investigation of iron deficiency anaemia, but should be considered if there are pointers in the history towards Crohn's disease.

5.19 Should I investigate my patient who has had a partial/total gastrectomy in whom I have discovered iron deficiency anaemia?

Iron (and B12) deficiency is very common in patients with a partial or total gastrectomy, probably because of the resultant hypochlorhydria (iron is absorbed best in an acid environment). These patients are, however, at an increased risk of developing gastric carcinoma 20 years after surgery.

The BSG recommends upper and lower gastrointestinal tract examination in such patients over 50 years of age.

5.20 One of my patients with longstanding coeliac disease has developed iron deficiency anaemia, having a previously normal full blood count on a gluten-free diet. Do they need investigating, or can I assume this is due to dietary indiscretion?

Iron deficiency anaemia is a common presenting feature of coeliac disease; however, this – together with other deficiencies (e.g. vitamin B12, folic acid) – should resolve on adoption of a strict gluten-free diet (and initial supplementation). If patients with coeliac disease subsequently develop iron deficiency, upper and lower gastrointestinal tract examination is warranted, bearing in mind the mildly increased risk of oesophageal, small bowel and colonic malignancy in this condition (Goddard et al 2000).

PATIENT QUESTIONS

5.21   Which foods are rich in iron?

Iron is best absorbed in its haem form – in other words, from red meats. Other good sources of iron (in descending order) include sardines, poultry, cod, wheat germ, lentils, soybeans, molasses and fortified breakfast cereals. Iron is best absorbed in its ferrous form, Fe^{2+}, which is soluble in water; however, most dietary iron is in the insoluble (at pH >3) ferric, Fe^{3+}, form, and is therefore best absorbed in an acidic environment (i.e. with vitamin C).

5.22   My doctor has prescribed iron tablets for me, but my next door neighbour told me that they cause constipation and I have stubborn bowels at the best of times. Is this true?

Most people tolerate iron tablets very well. There are several different preparations but there is little difference between them. They can cause indigestion, and some people find that they cause constipation. Occasionally they can cause diarrhoea in patients who have colitis (inflammation of the bowel). A few people are unable to tolerate any iron preparation by mouth, or do not respond to the medicine. In these cases, iron can be given as an infusion (via a drip as a day case in hospital). There is a very tiny risk of allergic reactions when iron is given this way, but fortunately it is very rare. Intramuscular injections tend to be painful and are therefore avoided.

Irritable bowel syndrome

6

6.1 What is irritable bowel syndrome?

Irritable bowel syndrome (IBS) is a functional gut disorder characterised by abdominal pain or discomfort with disturbed defaecation.

Attempts to define the condition more precisely in terms of symptom complex have been driven partly by the need to try to make IBS a positive diagnosis (rather than a diagnosis of exclusion), and also to define a more homogeneous group for trials.

The Rome II criteria (*Box 6.1*) are currently used to positively identify IBS, with exclusion of other conditions by appropriate investigations, depending on factors such as the patient's age and past medical or family history.

PREVALENCE, CAUSES AND INVESTIGATIONS

6.2 How common is irritable bowel syndrome?

IBS is extremely common. Studies vary but the overall prevalence is approximately 10% (range 4–22%). About 50% of people with functional gastrointestinal disorders (chiefly IBS and functional dyspepsia) consult their general practitioner, but only 20% of these are referred to secondary care in any given year.

BOX 6.1 Rome II diagnostic criteria for irritable bowel syndrome

At least 12 weeks, which need not be consecutive, in the preceding 12 months of abdominal discomfort or pain that has two of the three following features:

1. relieved with defaecation
2. associated with a change in frequency of stool
3. associated with a change in consistency of stool.

Symptoms that cumulatively support the diagnosis of irritable bowel syndrome include:

- abnormal stool frequency (for research purposes, 'abnormal' may be defined as more than three bowel movements per day or less than three bowel movements per week)
- abnormal stool form (lumpy/hard or loose/watery stool)
- abnormal stool passage (straining, urgency or feeling of incomplete evacuation)
- passage of mucus
- bloating or feeling of abdominal distension.

6.3 Does irritable bowel syndrome matter and what is its social impact?

Yes it does matter, both to the individual with the condition, and to society.

Symptoms of IBS may interfere with normal social activities and reduce quality of life. The US Householder Study (Drossman et al 1993) found that people with IBS miss almost three times as many days at work as those devoid of bowel symptoms (13.4 versus 4.9 days). It also revealed that IBS sufferers visited physicians 1.64 times for gastrointestinal complaints (compared to 0.09 for those without bowel symptoms) and were twice as likely to visit with non-gastrointestinal complaints (3.88 versus 1.77 times for those without bowel symptoms). Females with IBS are three times more likely to have a hysterectomy. In the US, the prevalence of IBS has been estimated at 15.4 million persons, and is associated with $1.6 billion in direct and $19.2 billion in indirect costs.

6.4 What causes irritable bowel syndrome?

There is no specific causative agent. There are proponents for psychological illness, abnormal illness behaviour, altered mood, autonomic reactivity and dysmotility. Others favour the hypothesis that a large proportion of patients with IBS have a food intolerance, which responds to exclusion of particular foods (Nanda et al 1989).

Patients with IBS constitute a heterogeneous group (even when tightly defined by the Rome criteria; *see Box 6.1*) and undoubtedly some fit into one or other of the above groups. The current favoured hypothesis is visceral hypersensitivity (*see Q 6.5*).

6.5 What is visceral hypersensitivity?

Visceral hypersensitivity describes the exaggerated awareness of 'normal' physiological processes in the gut.

IBS patients often complain that insufflation of air at rigid sigmoidoscopy reproduces their typical IBS pain. More formal studies have shown pain induced by much lower colorectal and small bowel balloon distension compared to control patients, despite somatic pain thresholds being higher in those with IBS.

6.6 What is 'spastic colon'?

This is a historical term for what we now consider – and more tightly define as – IBS.

6.7 Can food poisoning or gastroenteritis cause irritable bowel syndrome?

Yes. There is no doubt that a certain subgroup of patients with IBS have their condition triggered by an episode of infective gastroenteritis.

An association of IBS or 'spastic colon' with a bout of gastroenteritis was recognised over 40 years ago when Chaudhary and Truelove noted that 34/130 of their patients with 'irritable colon syndrome' dated the onset of their symptoms to a dysenteric illness.

More recently, a single small cohort of patients followed up 12 months after an outbreak of Salmonella food poisoning revealed that one-third had developed new IBS symptomatology (McKendrick & Read 1994). A large prospective cohort study confirmed this association, with 14 out of 318 (4.4%) culture-positive gastroenteritis patients developing IBS at 1 year follow-up, compared to 2027 out of 584 308 (0.3%) of the general population over the same time period, giving a relative risk of 11.9 (Rodriguez & Ruigomez 1999).

6.8 Can abnormal bacteria in the colon be responsible for irritable bowel syndrome?

This is not a well-studied area. The colon contains hundreds of species of bacteria, the vast majority of which are anaerobic. A single millilitre or gram of stool may contain 10^{12} bacteria. It is clear that alterations in flora may cause upset of normal physiology, for example:

- Antibiotic-associated diarrhoea occurs in up to 20% of recipients
- Pseudomembranous colitis due to colonisation of the bowel by *Clostridium difficile* can follow antibiotic therapy
- Functional diarrhoea/IBS may be triggered by an episode of food poisoning.

The most common commensal bacteria found in the colon are Bacteroides, Bifidobacteria, Lactobacilli, Clostridia, Enterococci, *Escherichia coli* and Staphylococci.

Renewed interest in the role of bacteria in the colon in both health and disease has led to the idea that ingestion of probiotics (Bifidobacteria, Lactobacilli, etc.) in commercially available 'yoghurt' drinks may be beneficial both in health and in certain disorders such as IBS. As yet there is no convincing evidence to substantiate these claims.

6.9 Is irritable bowel syndrome 'all in the mind'?

Psychiatric disorders (e.g. anxiety and depression) appear to occur more commonly in patients who present to their doctors with IBS. A prospective study looking at the development of IBS following an episode of gastroenteritis found that psychological disturbance at the time of the insult predicted the development of chronic IBS symptomatology (Gwee et al 1999) (*see also Q 6.18*).

6.10 How should I investigate irritable bowel syndrome?

Most studies on IBS have taken place in the secondary care setting, resulting in studies on a selected group who are perhaps less likely to accept a psychological explanation for their condition, believing there is an organic disease.

In the community, a diagnosis of IBS can usually be safely made on the basis of typical symptoms and a normal physical examination alone. Patients displaying any alarm features (e.g. anaemia, rectal bleeding, weight loss) or nocturnal symptoms should be investigated and/or referred to hospital as appropriate.

Patients under 45 years of age, with a long typical history (>2 years) and fluctuating symptoms probably have IBS. Female gender and frequent attendance with non-gastrointestinal symptoms (e.g. malaise, backache and urinary frequency) make the diagnosis more likely. Indeed, in the absence of alarm symptoms, the Rome II criteria have a specificity of over 98% for IBS, i.e. there is little chance of organic disease if the patient fulfils the criteria (Vanner et al 1999).

If the history is atypical or of short duration, the tests outlined in *Box 6.2* should be considered.

In a large secondary care study, 1452 IBS patients were tested for thyroid dysfunction and lactose intolerance, and had stool microscopy and fat examination, together with a flexible sigmoidoscopy and biopsy. Thyroid abnormalities were found in 6%, inflammatory bowel disease was detected in 1% and 21–25% had lactose intolerance (Hamm et al 1999).

BOX 6.2 Investigations in irritable bowel syndrome

- Full blood count (anaemia warrants investigation; raised platelet count may indicate chronic bleeding or suggest inflammatory bowel disease)
- Erythrocyte sedimentation rate
- Thyroid function tests (6% of 'IBS' patients show abnormalities)
- Anti-endomysial antibody/tissue transglutaminase (5% of 'IBS' patients have coeliac disease)
- Stool for microscopy and culture (? Giardia)
- Sigmoidoscopy

NB: Patients developing irritable bowel syndrome over the age of 45 should be referred for further investigation and will often require imaging of the bowel with either colonoscopy or a barium enema.

A recent case control study (300 Rome II criteria IBS patients and 300 healthy controls) has shown a 5% prevalence of coeliac disease in patients diagnosed with Rome II criteria IBS in the hospital setting (Sanders et al 2001). This is not surprising, given that coeliac disease can present with diarrhoea and bloating.

TREATMENT

6.11 How should I treat irritable bowel syndrome?

Treatment depends on the severity of the symptoms. Most patients are content with an explanation of the condition and reassurance that they are not suffering from a serious condition. It is important, however, to make a positive diagnosis and to listen to the concerns of the patient. Dietary or lifestyle changes may play a part in treatment (e.g. regular meals or avoidance of certain foods, stress management, etc.).

Some patients notice that certain foods make their symptoms worse and may avoid certain products (e.g. wheat, onions, chocolate) (Nanda et al 1989). An exclusion diet may be reasonable to try. This involves eating only rice and grilled chicken or steamed fish and drinking only water for 2–3 days to see if this alleviates symptoms and then adding in foods sequentially to identify those that trigger symptoms. The most common foods which are reported to exacerbate symptoms are wheat, dairy products (especially cheese, yoghurt and milk), coffee, potatoes, corn, onions, beef, oats and white wine. It is, however, important that patients avoid an unnecessarily restricted diet.

6.12 What drugs are useful in treating irritable bowel syndrome?

There are problems in both the design and interpretation of drug trials in IBS:

- previous lack of a precise definition led to heterogeneous patient study groups
- short length of studies (or treatment duration)
- fluctuating symptoms (exacerbate problems of short length of study)
- small studies
- high placebo response (40–70%), therefore difficult to conclusively prove that a drug is definitely having a beneficial effect per se
- lack of hard end points (morbidity, mortality).

In a recent review of randomised controlled trials in the treatment of IBS (Akehurst & Kaltenthaler 2001):

- 93 trials were identified (1987–98)
- only 45 were randomised

■ only six randomised controlled trials were deemed to provide adequate information.

6.13 Are bulking agents useful?

Yes, isphagula husk (Fybogel, Regulan) is of proven use. A double blind trial of Regulan tds for 12 weeks in 80 patients with IBS found 82% to gain overall improvement compared to 53% taking placebo. Unsurprisingly, constipation improved significantly (Prior & Whorwell 1987).

Bran may, however, make symptoms worse. In a double-blind, cross-over trial using 7 weeks of bran (12 g) versus placebo in 80 patients with IBS, there was no significant difference in improvement (52% versus 54%, respectively). Moreover, symptoms of wind were made worse by the bran (Snook & Shepherd 1994).

6.14 Is peppermint oil useful?

Probably not. Peppermint oil is a smooth muscle relaxant, and might reasonably be thought to help if spasm is important in IBS symptomatology. Although individual trials have shown benefit, a recent meta-analysis of eight trials failed to establish any significant benefit (Pittler & Ernst 1998).

6.15 Are other antispasmodics/anticholinergics useful?

Yes. In a meta-analysis of 26 double-blind trials, antispasmodics and anticholinergics have been shown to improve symptoms (drug 64% versus placebo 45%) (Poynard et al 1994). In this meta-analysis, mebeverine (Colofac) resulted in global improvement, but had no significant effect on pain. The best drugs for improving pain in IBS were cimetropium bromide (an anticholinergic which is not available in the UK) and dicyclomine hydrochloride (Merbentyl).

6.16 Are antidepressants useful in the treatment of irritable bowel syndrome?

Yes, for both global improvement and pain. Antidepressants work by altering visceral sensitivity, reducing central pain perception via an effect on the afferent nerves from the gut. They may also treat any associated psychiatric co-morbidity.

A meta-analysis of 11 trials using antidepressants for the treatment of functional gut disorders (eight IBS, two non-ulcer dyspepsia, and one studying both; Jackson et al 2000) showed an odds ratio for improvement of symptoms of 4.2 (95% CI, 2.3–7.9) with a number needed to treat (NNT) of 3. The analysis showed that there was a significant improvement in abdominal pain. Most of the trials ($n = 9$) used tricyclic antidepressants:

amitriptyline ($n = 3$), tramipramine ($n = 3$), desipramine ($n = 2$) and clomipramine ($n = 1$).

It is usual to start antidepressants at very low doses (e.g. amitriptyline 10–25 mg at night-time).

Tricyclic antidepressants (e.g. amitriptyline) may cause constipation and as such would be logically of more benefit in patients with diarrhoea-predominant IBS. Selective serotonin reuptake inhibitors (SSRIs; e.g. fluoxetine, citalopram) are increasingly used (and theoretically better for the constipation-predominant IBS group), although there are no published randomised controlled studies in IBS.

6.17 What is the role of 5-hydroxytryptamine (5-HT, serotonin) in the treatment of irritable bowel syndrome?

5-HT3 receptor antagonists

5-HT3 receptor antagonists have potential use in IBS. 5-HT3 receptors are widely distributed on visceral afferent nerves and enteric motor neurones. Antagonism reduces visceral pain.

Alosetron, a 5-HT3 receptor antagonist, significantly reduced pain and diarrhoea in female diarrhoea-predominant IBS patients (41% versus 29% placebo) over a 3-month period (Camilleri et al 2000). Unfortunately, the drug was withdrawn from the American market in November 2000 because of concerns about an association with ischaemic colitis, although it was re-approved by the Food and Drug Administration (FDA) for restricted use in Spring 2002.

5-HT4 partial agonists

5-HT4 partial agonists show promise for constipation-predominant IBS. Tegaserod has been shown to give global relief of IBS symptoms and constipation in constipation-predominant IBS patients (83% females) with a size effect of 10–14% (Mueller-Lissner et al 2000).

6.18 Is there any role for psychological treatment in irritable bowel syndrome?

Various psychological treatments have been tried in IBS, including:

- relaxation techniques
- hypnosis
- biofeedback
- cognitive behavioural therapy
- psychodynamic therapy.

However, most studies are generally flawed as there is no blinding and no effective placebo (many of the patients entering these trials have been tried on and failed many medical therapies, so to continue on medical therapy necessarily induces negative expectancy).

On the other hand, hypnotherapy has been reported to have dramatic effects (Whorwell et al 1984, 1987, Drugs and Therapeutics Bulletin 2005). In an early report just over 20 years ago (Whorwell et al 1984), 30 severely refractory IBS patients were randomised to either hypnotherapy or psychotherapy plus placebo medicine. Substantial improvements were seen in the hypnotherapy group at 3 months for abdominal pain, distension, bowel habit and wellbeing, and this was maintained at 2 years.

Constipation

7

7.1 What is constipation?

> Patients usually complain of constipation if they find defaecation difficult or pass stools infrequently. The Rome II criteria define constipation as at least 12 weeks per year of two or more of the following:
>
> ■ straining
> ■ lumpy or hard stool
> ■ sensation of incomplete evacuation
> ■ sensation of anorectal obstruction or blockage
> ■ fewer than three bowel movements per week.
>
> Clinically, more important than absolute frequency or consistency is a recent change in either parameter.

7.2 What is a normal bowel frequency?

Seventy per cent of those on a Western diet pass one stool per day; 95% of the population open their bowels between three times per day and three times per week.

7.3 How common is constipation?

In the UK, 1% of the population consult their family doctor annually, complaining of constipation, and 12 million GP prescriptions were written for laxatives in England in 2001 (Department of Health 2001). In surveys, 10–20% of people consider themselves to be constipated at some time (Thompson & Heaton 1980).

The prevalence of constipation increases with age. Up to a third of those over 65, particularly women, complain of constipation. Use of laxatives may be an accurate marker of the prevalence of constipation. About a fifth of people take laxatives occasionally, with 1 in 20 using laxatives weekly. Weekly, or more often, usage is far more prevalent in those aged over 65 (20–30%) (Thompson & Heaton 1980).

7.4 Is constipation linked to disease?

It is commonly supposed that constipation causes haemorrhoids. This is far from certain although constipation may cause haemorrhoidal bleeding or exacerbate anorectal discomfort in a patient with haemorrhoids.

Data on chronic constipation as a risk factor for colorectal cancer are again controversial. In particular, constipation may be a surrogate for other, more plausible risk factors (e.g. low dietary fibre, high cholesterol diet, etc.). However, a recent onset of constipation might be part of the change in bowel habit (it occurs rarely as an isolated symptom) that accompanies the presentation of a carcinoma.

Constipation can certainly cause stercoral (caused by mucosal irritation from hard constipated stool) ulceration and, rarely, even perforation. Constipation may also be causally linked to incontinence by excessive straining causing damage to the nerve supply of the urethral sphincter.

Finally, constipation cannot be said to be the cause of either diverticular disease or irritable bowel syndrome but may be an associated feature of either condition.

7.5   Which diseases may cause constipation?

Systemic diseases, disorders of the smooth muscle or the enteric nervous system of the colon, and disorders of the anorectum and pelvic floor may all cause constipation.

Systemic disorders

Hypothyroidism, diabetes mellitus (due to neurological effects) and hypercalcaemia (hyperparathyroidism, sarcoidosis and bony metastatic disease) may all cause constipation.

Multiple sclerosis and Parkinson's disease may be complicated by constipation, with immobility, drug side-effects and possibly depletion of dopaminergic nerves in the enteric nervous system all contributory to the latter.

Transection of the spinal cord and lesions of the sacral cord are often complicated by constipation.

Colonic smooth muscle disorders

Congenital and acquired colonic myopathies are extremely rare. They result in a hypotonic bowel with resultant pseudo-obstruction (see Q 7.13).

Systemic sclerosis (scleroderma) may cause fibrosis of the smooth muscle of the bowel.

Enteric nervous system disorders

Hirschsprung's disease is due to congenital absence or reduction in the myenteric ganglia, producing a functional obstruction (see Q 7.12).

Myenteric enteropathies may be acquired – for example, Chagas' disease which results from infection with Trypanosoma cruzi.

Occasionally the enteric nervous system can be affected as a paraneoplastic phenomenon, producing a paraneoplastic visceral neuropathy (e.g. small cell lung carcinoma).

Anorectal and pelvic floor disorders

A rectocele occurs when the rectovaginal wall bulges anteriorly into the vagina. Stool is then pushed into a blind-ended sac, and the patient may complain of difficulty evacuating stool, a lump in the introitus on straining, and may find that evacuation is not possible unless she pushes posteriorly on the rectovaginal septum to 'straighten out' the bulge.

A rectocele is demonstrated by a defaecating proctogram (*see* Q 13.23). Surgical repair may be beneficial in selected cases.

Weakness of the pelvic floor following traumatic childbirth may result in greater descent of the pelvic floor on straining and difficulty evacuating stool. This is termed the 'descending perineum syndrome'.

7.6 How should I investigate constipation?

It is essential to obtain a good history, and understand what the patient means when complaining of 'constipation'. It would seem prudent to check in all age groups:

- calcium (to exclude hypercalcaemia)
- thyroid function (to exclude hypothyroidism).

If the patient is young, there is no indication to image the bowel; however, in the older patient (>45 years old), most physicians would do so, unless the constipation was longstanding. A barium enema may seem preferable to a colonoscopy, since the likelihood of organic pathology is low and colonoscopy carries a small but definite risk of perforation.

Constipation as the only symptom is rarely the marker of serious disease, especially if longstanding.

7.7 How should I investigate constipation not responding to laxatives?

Young patients (in their twenties/thirties) should probably have a flexible sigmoidoscopy to exclude any distal pathology. A plain abdominal x-ray will identify occasional people with megarectum or megacolon (*see* Q 7.11). If plain abdominal x-ray is normal, a Shapes study (ingesting radio-opaque plastic pellets and measuring time to excretion) may be useful.

In older patients, examination of the colon is needed to exclude carcinoma (which may rarely present with isolated constipation) or a diverticular stricture. A barium enema is a reasonable investigation in this group, since a carcinoma or stricture large enough to cause constipation will be readily identified by this technique.

7.8 How should I manage/treat constipation?

It is important to ensure that the patient has good dietary intake of fibre, adequate fluid intake and engages in exercise, although evidence is lacking that any of these lifestyle measures is effective (Frizelle & Barclay 2004). Reassurance is sometimes all that is necessary, since often the patient worries that they should open their bowels daily and are concerned that a lesser frequency may predispose to illnesses. It is also important to review the drug history as several drugs may cause or exacerbate constipation (*Box 7.1*).

If simple measures do not improve the situation, then one or a combination of laxatives may be prescribed. There is little comparative data on the efficacy of many of the laxatives, although the purgatives used for bowel cleansing prior to colonoscopy or barium enema are clearly the most efficacious (Picolax, Kleenprep, Fleet, etc.).

There are no guidelines or protocols for the sequential use of laxatives. *Table 7.1* represents the approximate order used by the authors, together with the advantages and disadvantages of the various agents.

7.9 What drugs are potentially available in the future to treat constipation?

New serotonergic drugs are showing promise (*see Q 6.17*). Tegaserod, a partial 5-HT4 receptor agonist, has been shown to be useful in constipation-predominant irritable bowel syndrome (Prather et al 2000). Prucalopride, another 5-HT4 receptor agonist, has been shown to increase frequency and transit rate through the gut.

7.10 What other treatments are available to treat constipation?

Bowel training and biofeedback may be helpful in difficult cases but availability may be limited to specialist centres.

Colectomy may be necessary in a few patients with severe constipation refractory to all other treatments. Very careful selection is required.

7.11 What is megacolon/megarectum?

These are descriptive terms only, based on radiographic measurements of the width of the rectum or colon. They refer to dilatation of the colon and/or rectum in the absence of mechanical obstruction. Megacolon or

---

BOX 7.1 Drugs commonly predisposing to constipation

- Opiates
- Calcium channel antagonists (amlodipine, verapamil, nifedipine)
- Amitriptyline (and others with anticholinergic properties)
- Serotonin receptor antagonists
- Aluminium hydroxide
- Ferrous sulphate

TABLE 7.1 Sequential use of laxatives in the treatment of constipation

Agent*	Advantages	Disadvantages	Notes
Bulking agents Ispaghula husk (Fybogel, Regulan) *(likely to be beneficial)* Methylcellulose (Celevac) Sterculia (Normalcol) Bran	'Natural' fibre, cheap	May cause bloating (especially bran)	Fibre is broken down to short chain fatty acids (acetate, proprionate and butyrate). Butyrate is the preferred 'fuel' for the colonocyte While supplemental fibre is often used to treat irritable bowel, bran may cause worsening of bloating and pain in this group of patients
Osmotic agents Lactulose *(likely to be beneficial)* Liquid paraffin *(unknown efficacy)* Macrogols (polyethylene glycol, Kleenprep, Movicol) *(beneficial)*	Lactulose is cheap	Lactulose may cause bloating, and some patients find it unpleasant to taste	Movicol is a non-absorbable polyethylene glycol (PEG) and holds water inside the lumen of the bowel. Such PEG solutions have been shown to be more efficacious than lactulose (Attar et al 1999) Movicol is essentially the same as Kleenprep (common preparation used prior to barium enema/colonoscopy), but in lower dosage Kleenprep requires ingestion of 3–4 litres of water and so may be difficult for some patients
Stimulants Senna Docusate sodium (partially bulking/softening agent) Sodium picosulfate (Picolax)	Generally more efficacious than bulking agents; senna is cheap	Stimulants tend to cause crampy abdominal pain	Worries over long-term, regular use of senna (potentially causing aperistaltic bowel although little actual evidence exists to support this) Picolax should not be used if there is clinical suspicion of obstruction (theoretical risk of perforation)
Suppositories Glycerine *(unknown efficacy)* Bisacodyl	Glycerine suppositories are cheap	Patient acceptance/compliance	Glycerine acts as a mild irritant and stimulates rectal peristalsis

* Where evidence exists about the efficacy or otherwise of a particular drug, this is quoted in bracketed italics (Frizelle & Barclay 2004).

megarectum may be secondary to a variety of conditions – for example, Hirschsprung's disease (congenital megacolon), ulcerative colitis (toxic megacolon), intestinal pseudo-obstruction or any cause of constipation (e.g. hypothyroidism, Parkinson's disease).

It is important to distinguish between the congenital type (Hirschsprung's) and the acquired types, since surgery is necessary in the former, whereas medical management with disimpaction and subsequent bowel retraining and laxative use is first line management in the latter.

7.12 What is Hirschsprung's disease?

This is a rare congenital disorder usually presenting at birth. It is due to aganglionosis of the distal colon (usually the rectosigmoid colon), resulting in a non-relaxing narrow segment of bowel, thus causing obstruction. Barium enema will usually be sufficient to diagnose the condition, but occasionally full thickness biopsy of the rectum is necessary. Treatment is surgical.

7.13 What is chronic intestinal pseudo-obstruction?

Chronic intestinal pseudo-obstruction (CIPO) is characterised by ineffective propulsion of contents along the intestine, resulting in clinical (e.g. distension, vomiting) and radiographic (e.g. fluid levels) evidence of obstruction in the absence of any mechanical blockage (e.g. carcinoma, diverticular stricture). It is often associated with changes in the gut wall leading to dilatation of any region of the intestine (e.g. megaduodenum, megacolon; *see Q 7.11*).

CIPO may be due to primary disorders of the smooth muscle or myenteric plexus ('chronic idiopathic intestinal pseudo-obstruction' encompasses a large number of these rare primary disorders) or may be secondary (e.g. opiates, systemic sclerosis, hypothyroidism).

7.14 What is 'slow transit' constipation?

This describes a progressive reduction in transit rate around the whole of the colon, resulting in abdominal discomfort and infrequent (often painful) passage of hard stools. Defaecation may occur as infrequently as once every 2–3 weeks. It is almost exclusively seen in women and is not uncommon. Osmotic or bulking laxatives should be used primarily, with stimulants intermittently.

7.15 What is 'obstructed defaecation'?

Obstructed defaecation describes a sensation of incomplete evacuation (or tenesmus). It is important to exclude distal pathology (e.g. polyp, carcinoma) with a digital examination and flexible sigmoidoscopy.

Patients with this symptom will often strain excessively and this may cause mucosal prolapse or a 'solitary rectal ulcer'. Solitary rectal ulcer is caused by ischaemia of the prolapsed mucosa. This type of ulcer has typical histological findings and must be biopsied to exclude carcinoma or Crohn's disease.

Descending perineum syndrome (*see Q 7.5*) typically results in obstructed defaecation and may also be complicated by mucosal prolapse and rectal ulceration.

A sensation of incomplete evacuation is a common feature of irritable bowel syndrome.

PATIENT QUESTIONS

7.16 Do I need to open my bowels daily?

No. The vast majority of the population open their bowels anywhere between three times a day and once every three days. The most important thing is that you feel comfortable with your bowel habit and don't feel distended, or have to strain excessively, or find defaecation painful.

7.17 I have always been constipated, and I am worried that this may lead to bowel cancer. Is this true?

No – don't worry. There is no significantly increased risk of developing bowel cancer. Population studies have, however, shown that those consuming higher fibre diets (and who are therefore likely to have faster colonic transit rates) have a lower incidence of colorectal cancer (Burkitt et al 1972).

Diarrhoea

Diarrhoea is a very common complaint. In the UK there are many thousands of cases of acute diarrhoea per annum. Chronic diarrhoea may occur in up to 5% of the US population per year. Although the cause of acute diarrhoea is usually infective, the causes of chronic diarrhoea are many and diverse and therefore represent a considerable diagnostic challenge for the physician. Unfortunately, there is almost no evidence base on the investigation of diarrhoea, and management will therefore differ between different physicians.

8.1   What is diarrhoea?

It is important to define diarrhoea. Most patients recognise diarrhoea as the passage of liquid stool. This is due to non-bound (free) water. The consistency of stool may be difficult to describe subjectively and therefore many physicians use frequency of passage of stool as a surrogate marker, defining diarrhoea as the passage of more than three stools a day.

A careful history is essential, as some patients will use the term diarrhoea to describe the passage of small amounts of hard pellety stool four or five times in close succession in the mornings with associated abdominal pain (likely irritable bowel syndrome), whereas others with pure continence problems may complain of diarrhoea.

8.2   How is diarrhoea classified?

Classification of diarrhoea into different types is an attempt to help the physician narrow down the potential diagnoses, and therefore initiate more targeted investigations. There are several ways of classifying diarrhoea, and no single one is perfect. In reality, physicians tend to combine the various features to guide their management. Diarrhoea may be classified as follows:

- acute versus chronic
- osmotic versus secretory
- low volume versus high volume
- watery versus fatty versus inflammatory
- according to stool weight.

Acute versus chronic diarrhoea
Acute diarrhoea is usually defined as self-limiting and lasting less than 4 weeks. It is almost always due to an infective cause. Such infections (e.g. Campylobacter, Salmonella, Shigella, viral etc.) will often need no treatment; however, if the patient is unwell or has systemic symptoms, a short course of ciprofloxacin may be prescribed. A few infections may be prolonged and persistent, particularly giardiasis and amoebiasis. It is important therefore to ensure that stool cultures have been taken at some point in the course of investigation of chronic diarrhoea (>4 weeks).

Osmotic versus secretory diarrhoea

Osmotic diarrhoea is due to the presence of poorly or non-absorbable sugars or anions/cations in the stool. As the intestine is not able to maintain an osmotic gradient, these solutes retain or hold water (so that the osmolality of the stool water approaches that of the body osmolality), increasing the volume and fluidity of the stool. This forms the rationale for measuring the 'osmotic gap' of the stool water, which quantifies the contribution of electrolytes and non-electrolytes to water retention in the stool. Because the intestine is unable to maintain an osmotic gradient, the osmolality of stool water is the same as body osmolality (approximately 290 mOsm/kg). The osmotic gap is calculated as $290 - 2[(Na^+) + (K^+)]$. The multiplication of 2 takes account of the associated anions (e.g. chloride).

In secretory diarrhoea, excess sodium and potassium remain in the intestinal lumen as a result of either defective absorption or excess secretion. The excess sodium and potassium ions retain an amount of water within the lumen to keep the osmolality at around 290 mOsm/kg and the osmotic gap remains small (<50 mOsm/kg). An example of a pure (but extremely rare) secretory diarrhoea is a VIPoma.

Disaccharides, unlike monosaccharides, are non-absorbable and need to be broken down to their constituent monosaccharides. Lactose (glucose + galactose), which is present in large quantities in milk and cheese, is broken down by lactase. Lactase deficiency (either congenital or acquired) may therefore result in an osmotic diarrhoea (lactose intolerance). The osmotic gap here would be large (typically >125 mOsm/kg) as the malabsorbed lactose makes up a substantial proportion of the osmotically active solute in the stool water (thereby diminishing the relative contribution/concentration of Na^+/K^+). Lactase, sucrase and fructase deficiency, as well as ingestion of poorly absorbed cations (Mg, PO_4, SO_4) – which are the active ingredients of certain laxatives – may all cause an osmotic diarrhoea (and large osmotic gap).

Many diarrhoeal conditions have both osmotic and secretory contributions (e.g. inflammatory bowel disease).

Low volume versus high volume stools

The rectosigmoid colon acts as a reservoir for stool under normal conditions. Small, frequent, low volume, painful passage of stool suggests an inflammatory condition affecting this area. Typically, disorders of the small bowel result in large volume stool (hence the bulky, malodorous stool seen classically in coeliac disease).

Watery versus fatty versus inflammatory stool

Watery diarrhoea is usually secondary to inability to absorb water from either electrolyte secretion or malabsorption (secretory) or ingestion of a poorly absorbed substance (osmotic). Fatty diarrhoea (pale, oily, difficult to flush) is due to malabsorption of fat in the small intestine (mucosal disease or pancreatic exocrine insufficiency). Inflammatory diarrhoea is characterised by associated blood or pus in the stool.

Stool weight as a measure of diarrhoea
In difficult cases of diarrhoea, the physician may admit the patient to hospital and measure the weight of stool for 3 days on a normal diet and on the fourth day fasted. Normal stool weight is usually less than 200 g/day. Fasting results in reduced stool weight in osmotic diarrhoea (since the osmotically active substance is not ingested) but not in secretory diarrhoea.

8.3 How should I investigate chronic diarrhoea?

A detailed history is essential. In addition, acute diarrhoea must be distinguished from chronic diarrhoea, since an infective cause is much more likely in the former.

Frequency of stool is the usual means of assessing severity although this has limitations since a patient with proctitis only may pass small frequent stools, but they may be formed (as most of the colon is able to perform its usual function of water resorption) and stool weight may be near normal. Nocturnal diarrhoea is strongly suggestive of organic pathology. Fatty stool suggests small bowel or pancreatic pathology, whereas blood or pus suggests large bowel pathology.

Previous surgery (peptic ulcer surgery may result in blind loops – and subsequent bacterial overgrowth) should be noted, and certain drugs may cause diarrhoea (e.g. proton pump inhibitors, colchicines, digoxin toxicity). Sorbitol and mannitol, poorly absorbed sugars, may be found in 'sugar-free' chewing gums and may lead to diarrhoea. A history of mouth ulcers may point towards a diagnosis of inflammatory bowel disease or coeliac disease.

Physical examination may reveal clubbing (Crohn's disease, coeliac disease), tremor and tachycardia (hyperthyroidism) or hyperpigmentation (Addison's disease). It is important to note the presence or absence of distension, tenderness, masses (Crohn's, colonic carcinoma) and bowel sounds in the abdominal examination.

There are no data on the value of screening blood tests in chronic diarrhoea. It would, however, seem sensible to perform the investigations outlined in *Box 8.1* in the initial work-up. Further work-up of chronic diarrhoea is usually performed in secondary care, when the tests outlined in *Box 8.2* may be performed.

8.4 What are the commonest causes of chronic diarrhoea?

Common conditions presenting as chronic diarrhoea include irritable bowel syndrome, ulcerative colitis, Crohn's disease and coeliac disease.

BOX 8.1 Investigations in chronic diarrhoea (primary care)

Full blood count
- Anaemia
  — iron deficiency anaemia needs upper and lower gastrointestinal tract investigation
  — B12 deficiency may point to terminal ileal Crohn's disease (impaired absorption) or small bowel bacterial overgrowth (bacteria utilise B12 and synthesise folate)
  — B12/folate deficiency may indicate extensive Crohn's or coeliac disease (both may also cause iron deficiency as well)
- Thrombocytosis
  — raised platelets may be reactive to chronic blood loss
  — frequently raised in active Crohn's disease (may be regarded as an inflammatory marker in this context)

Biochemistry
- Raised urea may be relevant to the severity of the diarrhoea
- Hypocalcaemia suggests malabsorption: ? coeliac disease, ? extensive small bowel Crohn's disease
- Hypoalbuminaemia is a marker of disease activity
- Thyroid function: thyrotoxicosis may cause diarrhoea

Endomysial antibody
- Sensitivity 75–100%; specificity 95% for coeliac disease (if clinical suspicion is high for coeliac disease, duodenal biopsies should still be obtained as false negative in up to 25%)
- *Note:* test for immunoglobulin A at same time as deficiency occurs in 2–3% of coeliac disease patients and the antibody is IgA (therefore will be falsely negative in this percentage)
- Tissue transglutaminase antibodies (TTG) are employed in some centres – this is the autoantigen in coeliac disease. Sensitivity and specificity are similar to endomysial antibodies

Stool cultures
- Two samples increase sensitivity – mandatory in the setting of acute diarrhoea
- Should also be performed at some point in the presentation of chronic diarrhoea as conditions such as giardiasis may persist

Sigmoidoscopy
- Useful to inspect rectum and distal sigmoid colon – if normal, effectively excludes ulcerative colitis
- *Note:* inflammatory changes due to infection are indistinguishable from those due to inflammatory bowel disease

BOX 8.2 Investigations in chronic diarrhoea (secondary care)

Flexible sigmoidoscopy

- This allows visualisation of the left side of the colon (up to the splenic flexure/distal transverse colon) and also allows biopsy specimens to be obtained
- Ulcerative colitis presents with erythema, friability or frank ulceration and haemorrhage involving the rectum and spreading for a variable distance proximally
- Crohn's disease – deep ulceration, cobblestoning, skip lesions (patchy inflammation) – may also be evident
- Biopsy specimens may also diagnose microscopic colitis (lymphocytic or collagenous colitis) which is characterised by a macroscopically normal appearance but microscopic inflammation
- Melanosis coli (brownish pigmentation of the colonic mucosa) may be evident, indicating excess laxative ingestion over years
- It is a relatively simple test which does not usually require sedation and has a very low risk of perforation/complication (*see Q 13.3*)
- If there is no cause evident at flexible sigmoidoscopy and the patient is over 40 years old, it is probably wise to complete the examination of the colon with a barium enema (or colonoscopy)

Colonoscopy

- As above, but allows visualisation of, and biopsy specimens from, the whole colon and terminal ileum if indicated
- Its advantage is that it may pick up right-sided lesions (polyps, cancer, ileocaecal Crohn's disease) which would be missed by flexible sigmoidoscopy alone
- It is a more invasive test with a perforation risk of approximately 1:1000 for diagnostic evaluation. It usually requires sedation and is technically more difficult than a flexible sigmoidoscopy (*see Q 13.4*).

Gastroscopy

- To obtain duodenal biopsies for the diagnosis of coeliac disease (*see Q 13.7*)
- Biopsies necessary if endomysial antibody positive (to confirm disease) and may be performed even if endomysial antibody negative (if clinical suspicion high)

Small bowel meal

- May be performed earlier in investigation if small bowel Crohn's disease likely (right iliac fossa pain, diarrhoea and weight loss)
- Used chiefly to look for evidence of Crohn's disease, but may pick up small bowel diverticulae (predisposing to small bowel bacterial overgrowth) (*see Q 13.14*)

BOX 8.2 Investigations in chronic diarrhoea (secondary care)—cont'd

Pancreatic function
- Elevated 3-day faecal fat collection may suggest pancreatic disease (although may be elevated in mucosal disease)
- Faecal elastase-1 is a pancreatic enzyme which may be detected in a random stool sample. Sensitivity and specificity reported to be high
- PABA/pancreolauryl tests (*see Q 13.20*) rely on breakdown of an unabsorbable compound by pancreatic enzymes, rendering them absorbable and subsequently detectable in the urine

Breath tests
- Glucose hydrogen breath test (*see Q 13.18*) to seek small bowel bacterial overgrowth
- Lactose hydrogen breath test (*see Q 13.19*) to detect lactase deficiency (although exclusion of milk and milk products from the diet may be a simpler, pragmatic and cheaper alternative)

White cell scan
- Technetium-labelled white cells accumulate in areas of inflammation (*see Q 13.16*)
- May be used where inflammatory bowel disease (particularly Crohn's disease) is suspected, but conventional investigations have been negative

75SeHCAT
- Synthetic radiolabelled bile salt which is ingested (*see Q 13.17*)
- Gamma camera images at days 0 and 7 reveal how much is retained (enterohepatic circulation)
- Absence or very low percentage retention on day 7 indicates malabsorption of bile salts by the terminal ileum
- Causes include disease (Crohn's) or resection of terminal ileum, postcholecystectomy and idiopathic

Gut hormones
- Fasting blood sample required. Sent to specialist centres and often takes 6 weeks for results
- Incredibly rare causes of diarrhoea
  — gastrinomas causing hypergastrinaemia (Zollinger–Ellison syndrome) cause diarrhoea by excess acid production inactivating pancreatic enzymes
  — VIPomas cause profuse watery (secretory) diarrhoea (*be alert to this possible diagnosis if there is marked hypokalaemia*)

> **BOX 8.2 Investigations in chronic diarrhoea (secondary care)—*cont'd***
>
> **Admission**
> - Hospital admission to a planned investigation unit is occasionally necessary for difficult cases
> - Stools may be collected over a 3-day period to objectively assess frequency and measure stool weight
> - If stool weight excessive, fasting on day 4 may help distinguish between osmotic and secretory diarrhoea (see above)
> - Urine samples for a laxative screen could be usefully taken during stay if not performed earlier

IRRITABLE BOWEL SYNDROME

8.5 What is irritable bowel syndrome?

Irritable bowel syndrome (*see Ch. 6*) is characterised by abdominal pain and disordered bowel habit. Constipation or diarrhoea may predominate. The diagnosis should be a positive one, with as few investigations performed as possible, rather than a diagnosis of exclusion following exhaustive invasive tests. The Manning criteria, described almost 30 years ago, have been superseded by the Rome II criteria, and should help the physician make a positive diagnosis (*Box 8.3*).

The guidelines published recently by the British Society of Gastroenterology (Jones et al 2000) advocate this approach. Patients presenting with new onset of irritable bowel symptomatology over the age of 45, or with atypical or sinister symptoms (rectal bleeding, anaemia, weight loss, etc.), should be referred to secondary care for further evaluation. This will almost always entail a lower gastrointestinal tract evaluation.

ULCERATIVE COLITIS

8.6 What is ulcerative colitis and how common is it?

Ulcerative colitis is an inflammatory disorder of the colon of unknown aetiology involving the rectum and spreading for a variable extent proximally. It is characterised by relapse and remission, with the first attack most commonly occurring between the ages of 20 and 40 years. Its incidence is approximately 1 per 10 000 persons per year in the high-incidence areas including the USA, UK, Australia and Northern Europe, and its prevalence approximately 1 per 1000 of the population.

BOX 8.3 Diagnosis of irritable bowel syndrome: Manning and Rome II criteria

Manning criteria
- Abdominal pain relieved by defaecation
- Looser stools with onset of pain
- More frequent stools with the onset of pain
- Abdominal distension
- Passage of mucus in stools
- Sensation of incomplete evacuation

Rome II criteria
At least 12 weeks (which need not be consecutive) in the preceding 12 months of abdominal discomfort or pain with two out of three of the following features:
— relief by defaecation
— onset associated with a change in the frequency of stool
— onset associated with a change in the consistency (form) of stool
- Supportive (but not essential) features:
— abnormal stool frequency (<3 per week or >3 per day)
— abnormal stool form (lumpy/hard or loose/watery
— abnormal stool passage (urgency, straining or feeling of incomplete evacuation)
— passage of mucus
— bloating or feeling of abdominal distension

It is a disease of ex- and non-smokers. It affects the recto/rectosigmoid region in approximately 50%, the left side of the colon (up to the splenic flexure) in approximately 20–30%, and the entire colon (pan or total colitis) in 20%. The first presentation is often slow and insidious, but can be abrupt and severe.

The mainstays of treatment are the 5-aminosalicylates and steroids (orally or rectally) and azathioprine or 6-mercaptopurine. Severe attacks, marked by extreme frequency, systemic upset, anaemia and hypo-albuminaemia, result in emergency colectomy in 20–30% of such cases.

8.7 How is ulcerative colitis diagnosed?

The diagnosis depends on the clinical history, sigmoidoscopic or colonoscopic features (together with histological specimens), and the exclusion of infection (by stool culture). It is important to note that an infective colitis can be indistinguishable from idiopathic ulcerative colitis, both macro- and microscopically. Additionally, infection may coexist with a flare-up of ulcerative colitis, and in some cases appears to be a trigger for relapse. It is therefore mandatory to obtain a stool specimen in any 'flare-up' of colitis.

8.8 What is the strategy for treating ulcerative colitis?

Treatment strategies depend on both the severity and the extent of disease.

Severity

Assessment of the severity of an attack is usually made on the following parameters:

- stool frequency
- presence or absence of blood in the stool
- tachycardia
- fever
- estimations of haemoglobin, albumin and inflammatory markers (ESR, C-reactive protein or orosomucoids).

The original classification of Truelove and Witts over 50 years ago remains the benchmark by which to assess the severity of the attack (*Table 8.1*).

Extent

Extent should be determined by either flexible sigmoidoscopy or colonoscopy. The key question is whether disease is confined to the left-side of the colon (i.e. distal to the splenic flexure) or whether it extends more proximally (extensive, or total colitis if the whole colon is involved), and in this respect a flexible sigmoidoscopy is satisfactory.

8.9 How should distal colitis be treated?

Inflammation in the rectum alone (proctitis) is readily amenable to local, topical treatment with suppository preparations. Either steroid suppositories (e.g. prednisolone suppositories 5 mg bd pr) or 5-aminosalicylic acid

TABLE 8.1 Modified Truelove and Witts criteria for assessing severity of acute flare of ulcerative colitis

Feature	Mild	Moderate	Severe
Motions/24 hours	<4	4–6	>6
Rectal bleeding	Absent/small	Moderate	Large
Tachycardia	None	None	>90 bpm
Haemoglobin	>11 g/dl	10–11 g/dl	<10 g/dl
ESR	<30		>30
Temperature	<37°C		>37.8°C

suppositories (e.g. mesalazine suppositories 500 mg bd pr) may be used, either alone or in combination. Suppositories may be used in addition to oral 5-aminosalicylic acid formulations. If these measures fail, then it is usual to try a short course of oral steroids (e.g. prednisolone 30 mg od, reducing by 5 mg per week).

A similar strategy may be adopted with proctosigmoiditis or left-sided disease except that the suppositories are replaced with enema preparations (e.g. predfoam enema or mesalazine foam enema) as these have been shown in radiolabelled studies to propagate retrogradely as far as the splenic flexure. If patients suffer frequent relapses of distal colitis or are steroid dependent, then second line immunosuppression with azathioprine or 6-mercaptopurine may be employed.

It is not uncommon to find that patients with proctitis or proctosigmoiditis are constipated proximally. The patient when questioned may admit to the passage of hard stool, or a loaded right colon may be seen on a plain abdominal x-ray. Treatment with Fybogel may be helpful symptomatically for relief of the constipation, and anecdotally may help resolve the proctitis.

8.10 How should extensive or total (pan) colitis be treated?

As disease activity extends beyond the range of enema preparations, any significant flare-up requires systemic (oral) treatment. It would be usual to start with prednisolone 40 mg once daily, reducing by 5 mg per week to treat a flare-up. Studies over 50 years ago showed a dose–range effect, with prednisolone 40 mg/day providing greater benefit compared to 20 mg/day. Prednisolone 60 mg/day showed some additional benefit at the cost of greater side-effects. Occasionally, therefore, prednisolone 60 mg/day may be used in the outpatient setting if a patient has failed to respond to a conventional treatment dose and is well systemically and/or has social reasons not to be admitted to hospital for intravenous steroids. If an attack is severe (or fails to respond to outpatient treatment), then the patient should be admitted to hospital for intravenous steroids.

8.11 When is hospital admission indicated?

Patients with moderate to severe attacks of colitis not responding to oral steroids should be admitted to hospital. It is usual to commence patients on hydrocortisone 100 mg qds (equivalent to prednisolone 80 mg/day) for a period of 5–7 days. If there is no response (clinically and/or biochemically), colectomy is indicated (occurs in 20–30%). Intravenous ciclosporin may be used early during the admission (days 4–7) if there is no response to steroids.

The original small double-blind, placebo-controlled trial in the USA in 1994 showed that over 80% of steroid-unresponsive patients went into remission with ciclosporin (Lichtiger et al 1994). Subsequent experience has, however, shown that approximately 50% of such 'salvaged' patients end up with a colectomy over the next 12 months. Ciclosporin treatment is therefore best used as a bridge, allowing patients who have not had the opportunity to try second-line immunosuppressants such as azathioprine or 6-mercaptopurine (typically young patients with their first attack) the option to be controlled medically rather than undergo colectomy.

8.12 What are the principles of maintenance treatment?

Most patients (around 80%) have intermittent flare-ups of their disease. The interval between relapses varies from weeks to years. Maintenance treatment aims to reduce the relapse rate. The mainstay of maintenance treatment is the 5-aminosalicylates (5-ASAs). The original studies on sulfasalazine (5-aminosalicylic acid attached to a carrier moiety salazopyrin, and released by cleavage of the azo bond by colonic bacteria) demonstrated that it reduced the risk of relapse fourfold. This benefit is seen to extend beyond 3 years and so patients should probably be maintained indefinitely. This strategy is supported by data suggesting that long-term maintenance with 5-ASAs may reduce the risk of developing colorectal carcinoma.

 The newer 5-ASAs – mesalazine (Asacol, Pentasa), olsalazine and balsalazide – show similar efficacy but have fewer side-effects. Nephrotoxicity is reported (interstitial nephritis) and blood dyscrasia may rarely occur, and it is probably wise to check the full blood count and renal function, and dipstick the urine at 6-monthly intervals.

8.13 What is self-guided management?

Many patients with ulcerative colitis have intermittent mild or moderate exacerbations of their disease, which respond quickly to short courses of oral steroids or local enema treatment. Increased education, the introduction of inflammatory bowel disease nurse specialists and the availability of telephone advice have led to the concept that many patients may prefer to manage their disease themselves. Indeed, recent publications have shown fewer outpatient visits and greater patient satisfaction, without any increase in the primary care workload (Robinson et al 2001).

8.14 What is the recommended approach to surveillance of those at risk?

Extensive or total ulcerative colitis renders the patient at an increased risk of developing colonic carcinoma. The increased risk starts approximately 8–10 years from diagnosis, and it is for this reason that surveillance should be started from this point. The British Society of Gastroenterology has recently published guidelines recommending screening colonoscopy at 3-yearly intervals during the second decade from diagnosis, with more frequent surveillance in subsequent decades. Patients with left-sided disease are also at an increased risk of colorectal cancer, and surveillance is recommended starting 15 years after the onset of the disease.

8.15 What is the prognosis in ulcerative colitis?

Overall, mortality is approximately the same as in the general population. Severe attacks requiring admission to hospital will require an emergency colectomy in 20–30% of cases. Mortality from an acute severe attack is under 2% (including operative mortality).

Eighty per cent of patients with ulcerative colitis have intermittent relapses occurring at intervals of weeks to years. A small minority, 10–15%, have chronic continuous disease and usually require colectomy. A few patients present with an acute, severe, first attack resulting in urgent colectomy.

8.16 What does the future hold for those suffering from ulcerative colitis?

It is likely that guided self-management will become more established in the future. The recent discovery of the IBD locus and NOD-2 gene, which has an important role in the predisposition to Crohn's disease, should provide further insight into the pathophysiology of the disease and allow development of more targeted therapy.

CROHN'S DISEASE

8.17 What is Crohn's disease and how common is it?

Crohn's disease is an inflammatory disorder of unknown aetiology affecting the gastrointestinal tract anywhere from the lips to the anus. It may be discontinuous (skip lesions) and is characterised by periods of relapse and remission. Strictures and fistulae are common complications. It has a predilection for the ileocaecal region, with approximately 50% of all patients with this distribution of disease. The colon alone is affected in approximately 20% of patients.

It is less common than ulcerative colitis, with incidence rates of 0.1 to 1 per 10 000 of the populations in North America, Europe and Australia. Unlike ulcerative colitis, there is a much higher prevalence in smokers. Antibiotics, 5-aminosalicylates, steroids, azathioprine or 6-mercaptopurine, methotrexate, infliximab and surgery may have important contributions in the management of the disease.

8.18 How is Crohn's disease diagnosed?

Diagnosis is made by a combination of clinical history, examination and blood tests, together with radiographic studies and endoscopy.

Although a history of diarrhoea, weight loss and right iliac fossa discomfort may be suggestive of Crohn's disease, a small bowel meal and ideally histology from ileocolonic biopsies obtained at colonoscopy are required to make the diagnosis. Crohn's disease presenting with vague abdominal pains and intermittent diarrhoea may be mistaken for irritable bowel syndrome.

A normal C-reactive protein and ESR make a diagnosis of Crohn's disease less likely. The platelet count should be noted as this is often elevated in active Crohn's disease.

Abdominal ultrasound or CT scanning may be particularly useful if an inflammatory mass or abscess is suspected.

8.19 What effect does smoking have in Crohn's disease?

Crohn's disease is much more prevalent among smokers, and smokers with Crohn's disease have more aggressive disease which is more likely to relapse and need surgical intervention.

It is very important that patients stop smoking. Evidence shows that successful cessation of smoking is associated with a better prognosis, particularly in females after surgical resection.

8.20 Which drugs are useful in the treatment of Crohn's disease?

Aminosalicylates

Aminosalicylates (5-ASAs) are frequently used in the treatment of Crohn's disease, although the data are conflicting. A large study showed benefit of mesalazine (Pentasa) 4 g/day over placebo in the treatment of mild to moderatly active Crohn's disease (Singleton et al 1993), but other studies have not found any benefit. Sulfasalazine, in doses of 4–6 g/day, may be useful in inducing remission in colonic Crohn's disease.

Evidence for the efficacy of 5-ASAs in the maintenance of Crohn's disease is weak. A meta-analysis by Camma and colleagues (1997) of over 2000 Crohn's disease patients demonstrated a modest benefit in maintenance of remission following surgical resection (absolute risk reduction 13%), but a more recent prospective trial assessing mesalazine in postsurgical resection patients failed to show any benefit (Lochs et al 2000).

Corticosteroids

Steroids are efficacious in the treatment of active Crohn's disease, with approximately 70% of patients entering remission on prednisolone 40–60 mg/day tapered over 6–12 weeks.

Thiopurines

Azathioprine and 6-mercaptopurine (thiopurines) have definite roles, both in terms of treatment of active disease (odds ratio = 3.1 over placebo, although they take 6–12 weeks to exert their effects) and in maintenance of remission (odds ratio = 2.3). They should be considered in steroid-dependent patients or those who fail to taper a second course of steroids occurring shortly after treatment of a first flare. There is a dosage effect, with the higher doses more effective. The target dose for azathioprine is 2.0–2.5 mg/kg/day and for 6-mercaptopurine 1.0–1.5 mg/kg/day.

 The thiopurines are generally well tolerated, but can have serious side-effects. Patients must be warned about potential symptoms or signs indicating excessive immunosuppression and also the small risk of pancreatitis. Frequent monitoring of bloods during the first few months of therapy is necessary (see Ch. 14).

Methotrexate

In those patients in whom azathioprine or 6-mercaptopurine either fails to maintain remission satisfactorily, or in those who are intolerant, methotrexate should be considered. A double-blind randomised controlled trial showed that 39% of steroid-dependent Crohn's disease patients given 25 mg methotrexate intramuscularly once per week entered remission and were able to withdraw completely from steroids, compared to just 19% receiving placebo (Feagan et al 1995). It is also beneficial in maintaining remission. The cohort of patients going into remission in the aforementioned trial were then randomised to either 15 mg methotrexate intramuscularly once per week or placebo. After 40 weeks of treatment, 65% of the methotrexate group were still in remission compared to 39% given placebo (Feagan et al 2000).

Methotrexate is given intramuscularly as its bioavailability is unpredictable when given orally. It is highly teratogenic, and so highly effective contraception should be used by women of child-bearing age.

Infliximab

Infliximab, an anti-tumour necrosis factor antibody, is a recently introduced and highly effective treatment for Crohn's disease. At a dose of 5 mg/kg as an intravenous infusion it has been shown to improve symptoms in 81% of patients with moderate to severe Crohn's disease versus 17% given placebo (Targan et al 1997). It is also effective in maintenance of remission by repeated infusions at 8 week intervals. It is, however, extremely expensive (currently over £1000 per infusion), antibodies may form and therefore render it less efficacious with repeated dosing, and it may reactivate tuberculosis. Obviously long-term side-effects are currently unknown.

Antibiotics

Antibiotics, such as metronidazole, have a role in the treatment of pyogenic complications of Crohn's disease. Metronidazole is often used in patients with colonic and perianal disease, and may be beneficial in healing simple perianal fistulae. Some data suggest that ciprofloxacin may also confer beneficial effects in active Crohn's disease.

8.21 Is diet important in the treatment of Crohn's disease?

Elemental and polymeric diets seem to be useful in inducing remission in Crohn's disease. They may be favoured over steroids in the treatment of children, or those with relative contraindications (e.g. severe osteoporosis) or intolerance of steroids. Compliance may, however, be an issue, as no other foods are allowed during the treatment periods which may be 6 weeks or more. There is a tendency to relapse once a conventional diet is adopted again.

8.22 What is the prognosis in Crohn's disease?

Data from the National Co-operative Crohn's Disease Study show that 78% of patients will have undergone surgery for their disease at 20 years from diagnosis (Mekhjian et al 1979).

Ileocaecal disease is most likely (and colonic disease least likely) to require surgical intervention. Although surgical resection of disease may afford many years without symptoms, 20–30% of patients will have a symptomatic recurrence within a year, with a further 10% of the remainder per year thereafter relapsing. Mortality rates are modestly elevated compared to the general population.

8.23 What is the recommended approach to surveillance of those at risk?

Patients with pan-colonic Crohn's disease have approximately the same degree of risk of developing colorectal carcinoma as patients with pan-colonic ulcerative colitis and should therefore be offered surveillance colonoscopy.

8.24 What does the future hold for those suffering from Crohn's disease?

Advances in the understanding of the genetics of Crohn's disease (e.g. NOD-2 gene) and the further development of biological agents (e.g. anti-adhesion molecule antibodies, interleukin antibodies) are likely to give better disease control in the future.

COELIAC DISEASE

8.25 What is coeliac disease and how common is it?

Coeliac disease is a gluten-sensitive enteropathy affecting the small bowel, which almost always responds clinically and histologically to withdrawal of gluten from the diet.

Over the last decade, with the introduction of serological assays (anti-gliadin, anti-endomysial and tissue transglutaminase antibodies), it has become clear that coeliac disease is much more prevalent than previously thought. Textbooks have quoted prevalence figures of around 1 in 2000 for the UK and Northern Europe, but it is now clear from serological testing of blood bank specimens that this figure is between 1 in 100 and 1 in 250.

The vast majority of adult patients do not complain of the classic symptoms of steatorrhoea and weight loss (classic coeliac disease), but rather present with iron deficiency anaemia, osteoporosis, abnormal liver function tests or even neurological symptoms (atypical coeliac disease).

8.26 How is coeliac disease diagnosed?

The gold standard for diagnosis remains the small bowel biopsy, which may be obtained via duodenal biopsies at gastroscopy. Classically, this shows subtotal villous atrophy with crypt hyperplasia, lymphocytic infiltration of the lamina propria and the presence of intraepithelial lymphocytes. Repeat duodenal biopsies are often obtained 6–12 months after the introduction of a gluten-free diet to document resolution of the subtotal villous atrophy; however, some physicians may be happy with a previous positive antibody test turning negative in association with resolution of the presenting complaint.

8.27 How is coeliac disease treated?

Patients should adopt a strict gluten-free diet for life. The majority, up to 90%, will improve clinically, biochemically and histologically. If the patient fails to respond to a gluten-free diet, or relapses following initial improvement, inadvertent ingestion of gluten should be suspected in the first instance and review by a dietitian is appropriate.

If the diet is adhered to strictly and there remains no response, other conditions which may cause subtotal or total villous atrophy should be sought, and coexisting conditions should be excluded (*Box 8.4*). If these causes are excluded, then the diagnosis is of refractory sprue (intractable coeliac sprue). This condition is rare, but may progress to ulcerative jejunoileitis and lymphoma. Recent evidence suggests that refractory sprue, ulcerative jejunoileitis and lymphoma are linked conditions, related to a

---

BOX 8.4 Alternative causes and diagnoses in villous atrophy

Other causes of villous atrophy
- Giardiasis
- Small bowel bacterial overgrowth
- Hypogammaglobulinaemia
- Post-gastroenteritis
- Tropical sprue

Other diagnoses to consider
- Irritable bowel syndrome
- Lactose intolerance
- Pancreatic insufficiency

---

clonal expansion of intraepithelial lymphocytes. Refractory sprue may respond to steroids or other immunosuppressive therapy.

Overt nutritional deficiencies (e.g. iron, folate, vitamin B12, calcium, magnesium, etc.) should be treated.

8.28 What is the prognosis in coeliac disease?

The prognosis is excellent for patients who adhere to a life-long, gluten-free diet. There is an approximately twofold greater incidence of malignant disease in adult coeliac patients compared to the general population. Small intestinal lymphoma is the most common of these, but there is also an increase in adenocarcinoma of the oesophagus, small intestine and colon. The small increased risk of malignant complications is probably reversed by adherence to a strict gluten-free diet.

8.29 How frequently should patients with coeliac disease be followed up?

Patients who remain well on a gluten-free diet need infrequent follow-up. It is probably wise to check a full blood count and possibly haematinics annually. This may be done in primary care or in a nurse/dietitian-led specialty clinic.

PATIENT QUESTIONS

8.30 Are there any dietary restrictions in ulcerative colitis?

There are no restrictions on diet. There are no foods that adversely affect the disease, nor is there evidence for any particular foods being beneficial.

Patients should, however, avoid non-steroidal anti-inflammatory drugs (NSAIDs) – for example, ibuprofen or diclofenac – as there is evidence that these increase the risk of a relapse.

8.31 Will I have to have my bowel removed?

No, the majority of patients with ulcerative colitis will not need a colectomy. Studies show that up to a third of all patients will undergo a colectomy at some point in the natural history of their disease. The greatest risk is for the first attack, if it is a severe colitis affecting the whole colon. Resection is required in 20–30% of such patients. If the first severe attack is controlled medically, the colectomy rate thereafter falls dramatically.

8.32 Is Crohn's disease curable?

Although a small proportion of Crohn's disease patients will present with an index attack of the disease and never have another flare-up, or alternatively have surgery to remove an affected segment of bowel and subsequently enjoy many symptom-free years, the majority of patients will have intermittent relapses of their disease. It should therefore be regarded as a chronic condition, although many patients are well controlled and have a very good quality of life.

8.33 What causes Crohn's disease?

This is currently unknown. There are many theories, including infectious agents (including *Mycobacterium paratuberculosis* – a bacterium related to the tuberculosis bacteria), refined sugars, toothpaste and abnormal leakiness of the bowel wall (permeability). Crohn's disease is also more prevalent amongst smokers. Genetic predisposition is an important factor, with first degree relatives of an affected person having approximately a 1 in 10 chance of developing the disease.

8.34 Are there any particular foods I should avoid (or try to eat) in coping with Crohn's disease?

No. You can eat anything you like. No foods have been shown to be beneficial or detrimental to the disease itself. If you have a stricture or narrowing of the bowel, particularly involving the small intestine, you may find that fibrous food (e.g. fruit and vegetables) causes stomach ache. This is because cellulose (the major part of fruit and vegetables) is non-digestible and may impact in front of a stricture. The bowel behind then squeezes (peristalsis) to try to force the lump of food through the narrowing and it is this that gives rise to the colicky pain. The pain disappears once the food successfully passes beyond the stricture. It doesn't actually aggravate the inflammation, but it can cause a lot of pain and discomfort. Such patients often find a low fibre (or low residue) diet helpful. Sometimes an operation may be necessary to either remove the short piece of bowel containing the stricture, or alternatively to open up the stricture.

8.35 In managing coeliac disease, do I just need to avoid wheat and wheat products?

No, barley and rye also need to be avoided (and therefore beer) since they contain a related group of proteins which are similar to gluten and appear to be toxic to the small bowel lining. Oats should be excluded initially on commencement of a gluten-free diet, until remission is achieved. It is apparent, however, that many patients with coeliac disease can in fact tolerate small amounts (up to 2 oz/day) of oat cereal, without any deleterious effect on clinical symptoms or duodenal histology, and so oats from a reliable source may be introduced at a later stage if desired and tolerated.

8.36 Do coeliacs need to stay on a gluten-free diet for the rest of their lives?

Yes. A small percentage of children with coeliac disease seem to become tolerant to gluten in adolescence (with normal small bowel histology), but coeliac disease diagnosed in adulthood should be considered life-long.

8.37 Are my children also likely to suffer from coeliac disease?

There is a genetic component to coeliac disease and there is a 1 in 10 chance that the offspring of an affected parent will develop the condition.

PATIENT QUESTIONS

Rectal bleeding and bowel cancer

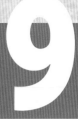

RECTAL BLEEDING

BOWEL CANCER

MANAGEMENT OF RECTAL BLEEDING

RECTAL BLEEDING

9.1 How common is rectal bleeding?

Rectal bleeding is a very common symptom in primary care and 80% of such patients do not seek medical advice (Crossland & Jones 1995). The risk of bowel cancer in patients presenting with rectal bleeding varies enormously according to the clinical setting – from 1:700 in the community to 1:30 in primary care to 1:16 in a hospital surgical clinic (Thompson et al 2003). Given that rectal bleeding is very much more common than bowel cancer, 2-week wait guidelines (*Box 9.1*) were introduced to facilitate effective referral patterns. There is some evidence that these guidelines are having an impact on referral patterns but less evidence that they are changing outcome for affected patients (Flashman et al 2004).

9.2 What are the different types of rectal bleeding?

The volume and type of bleeding can vary enormously. Clinically, different types of bleeding can be classified but the usefulness of this in practice is unproven. Blood may be:

- bright red, coating the stool or splashing in the pan/only on toilet paper: suggests local or anal causes
- bright red, mixed in with normal stool: suggests colorectal neoplasia
- bright red with diarrhoea: chronically suggests inflammatory bowel disease; acutely suggests infection or diverticular bleeding
- darker blood: suggests proximal neoplasia or ischaemic colitis
- melaena: suggests bleeding proximal to the hepatic flexure.

Torrential lower gastrointestinal haemorrhage (i.e. enough to cause haemodynamic instability) is rare. It is important to exclude upper

---

BOX 9.1 Criteria for 2-week referral for patients with suspected bowel cancer

1. Rectal bleeding with a change in bowel habit to loose stools and/or increased frequency of defaecation persistent for 6 weeks; all ages
2. Change in bowel habit as above, no rectal bleeding but age >60 years
3. Rectal bleeding without anal symptoms; age >60 years
4. Right-sided palpable mass; all ages
5. Definite (not pelvic) rectal mass; all ages
6. Unexplained iron deficiency anaemia; men all ages, postmenopausal women

Data from Thompson et al 2003.

gastrointestinal causes first (with endoscopy), then proceed to lower gastrointestinal investigation (*see Q 9.3*). Cancer rarely causes torrential bleeding; diverticular disease or vascular abnormalities are more common causes in this clinical setting. However, the accuracy of experienced clinicians' or patients' estimation of faecal blood loss is poor, thus making such information unhelpful apart from generalisations such as 'torrential'.

9.3 Which patients with rectal bleeding should be investigated and how?

Bright red rectal bleeding, separate to the stool and with an obvious rectal or anal cause (e.g. prolapsing haemorrhoids, history suggesting an anal fissure), is highly unlikely to suggest underlying neoplastic pathology, especially in patients under 50 years of age. Likewise, rectal bleeding associated with constipation is unlikely to be significant. In contrast, recurrent gastrointestinal bleeding with diarrhoea or alternating bowel habit, or blood mixed with the stool and no obvious anal cause, are more sinister symptoms and deserve urgent referral to secondary care (*see Box 9.1*) The 2-week wait referral for lower gastrointestinal malignancy is based on these premises.

The minimum investigation that any patient with rectal bleeding should undergo is an inspection of the anus and a rectal examination. In those in whom further investigation is deemed necessary, either a flexible sigmoidoscopy ± barium enema or a colonoscopy should be offered.

9.4 What factors determine when a barium enema is indicated?

The authors believe that older strategies, such as rigid sigmoidoscopy with or without completion barium enema, are no longer appropriate unless the clinical presentation is entirely benign and a clear anorectal cause is discovered at rectal examination/proctoscopy/rigid sigmoidoscopy (*see Qs 13.1 and 13.2*).

Rectal bleeding should be investigated with flexible endoscopy. It is not clear whether this should be flexible sigmoidoscopy (easier bowel preparation, less patient discomfort and, perhaps, less risk; *see Q 13.3*) or colonoscopy (more complete examination, more complicated bowel preparation, potentially more complications, more likely to need sedation; *see Q 13.4*).

The final choice of investigation strategy will depend on local expertise and availability, as well as the patient's clinical presentation. Any patient whose initial investigation shows a left-sided (distal to splenic flexure) lesion (polyp or cancer) will need a complete colonic examination in due course. Patients at higher risk of colorectal neoplasia are best investigated with colonoscopy.

9.5 How should torrential gastrointestinal bleeding be investigated?

Patients should first be resuscitated. Gastroscopy is often performed to exclude an upper gastrointestinal cause of haemorrhage. Colonoscopy is often difficult in this clinical setting because of poor preparation and poor views. A skilled, experienced colonoscopist can sometimes, with careful technique, evaluate the cause of torrential lower gastrointestinal tract bleeding and may even offer therapy (e.g. clipping a bleeding diverticular artery, cauterising an area of vascular ectasia).

The mainstay of the investigation of torrential gastrointestinal bleeding without obvious cause is angiography. This allows accurate identification of a bleeding point and allows targeted radiological or surgical intervention. Unfortunately, relatively rapid blood loss is needed for angiography to detect the bleeding point.

9.6 What causes rectal bleeding?

Common causes of rectal bleeding include:

- haemorrhoids
- anal fissure
- ulcerative colitis
- colorectal neoplasia
- bacterial infections.

Less common causes include:

- Crohn's disease
- ischaemic colitis
- solitary rectal ulcer
- diverticular disease
- vascular malformations.

BOWEL CANCER

9.7 What causes bowel cancer?

A small proportion (<5%) of colorectal cancer (CRC) is caused by defined genetically inherited polyposis syndromes, i.e. familial adenomatous polyposis (FAP) and hereditary non-polyposis colorectal cancer (HNPCC). Other conditions that predispose to the development of CRC include extensive inflammatory bowel disease (either ulcerative colitis or Crohn's disease, especially in association with primary sclerosing cholangitis) and ureteric drainage into the bowel. However, the vast majority of bowel cancer arises de novo from sporadic polyps.

Why some patients develop polyps and why only some polyps (around 10%) undergo invasive malignant change is not clearly understood. Factors include genetic influences and diet (excess red meat and deficient dietary fibre may increase risk).

9.8 How common is bowel cancer?

Bowel cancer is the second most common cause of cancer death in the UK (second to bronchus), with a lifetime incidence of 2–3%, causing up to 20 000 deaths per year in the UK (16% of cancer deaths). Most cancers are still left-sided (between the splenic flexure and rectum) but there seems to be a relative increase in the incidence of right-sided neoplasia (from caecum to splenic flexure) (*Box 9.2*).

Up to 50% of colorectal neoplasia may be detected by simple rigid sigmoidoscopy but synchronous tumours (i.e. tumours in more than one site at the same time) occur in up to 10% of patients so the detection of a distal neoplasm should always lead to an examination of the whole bowel (postoperatively in the case of an obstructing distal tumour).

9.9 How is bowel cancer treated? What percentage of bowel cancer patients need a colostomy?

The primary treatment for bowel cancer is surgical resection. The exact type of operation performed depends on the anatomical location and stage of the tumour. Caecal, ascending and transverse colonic tumours are treated with a right hemicolectomy, usually with a primary anastomosis (performed at the time of initial surgery). Left-sided tumours (the majority) are treated with anterior resection and primary anastomosis, or – if too near to the anus to preserve sphincteric function – with abdominoperineal resection with the formation of a permanent stoma or colostomy and excision of the entire rectum.

Apart from during abdominoperineal excisions, the formation of a temporary stoma may be necessary in the other types of operation. Factors that make this more likely include emergency surgery, particularly in those patients presenting with obstruction or coexisting co-morbidity.

BOX 9.2 Incidence of right-sided neoplasia

Anatomical site	Percentage of cases
Rectum	40
Sigmoid and descending colon	25
Transverse colon	10
Caecum and ascending colon	25

Patients with isolated liver or lung metastases may also be treated surgically, occasionally after preoperative downstaging with chemotherapy. Patients with favourable liver metastases status (fewer than three, unilobar, all <3 cm) have up to a 40% 5-year survival rate after liver resection surgery.

9.10 What role does chemotherapy play in the treatment of bowel cancer?

Chemotherapy is increasingly used in the treatment of patients with bowel cancer. It may be used as an adjunct to surgery in an attempt to improve the chances of cure or as palliative therapy in those either unfit for surgery or with postsurgical recurrence (*see Ch. 15*).

9.11 What role does radiotherapy play?

Radiotherapy has a limited role as an adjunctive treatment in those with rectal cancer or as a device to 'down-stage' such patients preoperatively.

9.12 What is the chance of cure from bowel cancer?

Cure from bowel cancer depends on the stage of the disease at presentation (*Table 9.1*): 55% of patients have Dukes stage C or D at diagnosis and hence limited survival. This fact is driving current strategies for population screening. (It should be noted that some experts use the TNM (tumour–node–metastasis) classification in preference to the original Dukes staging system, as outlined in *Table 15.1*.)

TABLE 9.1 Staging of bowel cancer

Dukes stage (modified)	Definition	Approximate frequency at diagnosis (%)	5-year survival rate (%)
A	Localised within bowel wall	11	83
B	Penetrating bowel wall	35	64
C	Lymph nodes	26	38
D	Distant metastases (usually liver)	29	3*

Source: Improving outcomes in colorectal cancer, Department of Health 1997.
* A minority of selected cases are suitable for hepatic resection, conferring a better survival rate.

9.13 Who needs referring to a family history clinic because of a family history of bowel cancer?

Familial adenomatous polyposis and its variants, juvenile polyposis and Peutz–Jegher, hereditary non-polyposis colorectal carcinoma (HNPCC), and patients with either young relatives or multiple relatives affected by colorectal carcinoma, should be referred to a family history clinic (*see Q 12.19* and *Table 12.1*).

9.14 What about mass screening for bowel cancer?

Mass population screening for bowel cancer is an integral part of current public health plans. The exact strategy is still under debate but options include faecal occult blood testing followed by colonoscopy for positive results or flexible sigmoidoscopy for all at age 50 (*see Ch. 12 for more details*).

The main problem with bowel cancer screening using endoscopic techniques is the complication rate. Approximately 1:1000 colonoscopies will be complicated by perforation or haemorrhage – either of which may be life-threatening (mortality rate 1:15 000–20 000). Contrast this with virtually zero complication rates of similar screening programmes such as for breast or cervical cancer.

MANAGEMENT OF RECTAL BLEEDING

9.15 What is the management of diverticular disease?

Diverticular disease is very common in middle-aged and elderly Western patients (50% in those aged over 50 in the Western world). The aetiology is unknown but is likely to be environmental as non-Western populations have a low incidence which then rises on settlement to a high risk area. Likely influential candidates in the aetiology include a low fibre diet in childhood.

Diverticular haemorrhage, although rare, can frequently be torrential (*see Q 9.5*). Most patients settle with transfusion and conservative management; others need urgent surgery following resuscitation.

Most episodes of acute diverticular inflammation or diverticulitis are best managed with antibiotics (perimural microabscess formation is well recognised). Recurrent episodes, or complications such as perforation or stricture formation, as well as acute torrential haemorrhage, are other indications for surgery.

The evidence base for either medical or surgical management in acute diverticulitis is limited (Simpson & Spiller 2004). Early studies have suggested that rifaximin, a rifampicin-like antibiotic, may reduce symptoms in chronic diverticulosis but further studies are needed before its widespread use can be advocated (Simpson & Spiller 2004).

9.16 How is the diagnosis of diverticular inflammation best made?

Diverticular inflammation usually presents with the triad of left iliac fossa pain, pyrexia and acute change in bowel habit in a patient with previously known or suspected diverticular disease. The first such attack may need hospital admission, where CT scan can help confirm the diagnosis acutely followed by colonoscopy or barium studies as an outpatient, assuming the acute attack settles. Subsequent attacks, assuming no systemic collapse or torrential bleeding, can often be managed conservatively with broad spectrum antibiotics and bed rest.

9.17 Which infections cause rectal bleeding?

Infection rarely causes isolated rectal bleeding without diarrhoea. Patients present with an acute diarrhoeal illness, often associated with abdominal cramps and fever. Bacterial suspects include Campylobacter, Salmonella and Shigella. Viral causes rarely cause blood per rectum as part of the clinical presentation.

9.18 What are the local or anal causes of rectal bleeding?

Haemorrhoids

These usually present as fresh blood without diarrhoea, splashing in the toilet pan or on toilet paper. Occasionally the patient may feel them as a lump 'coming down'.

- ■ *Diagnosed by*: proctoscopy (*Fig. 9.1*) (*see also Q 13.1*). *Note:* PR examination will often be normal in patients with haemorrhoids.
- ■ *Treatment*: Proctasydyl ointments, Anusol. Banding and sclerotherapy performed in the surgical outpatient clinic.

Anal fissure

This is characterised by intense pain on defaecation, and is often associated with constipation.

- ■ *Diagnosis*: often diagnosed on the clinical history. Rectal examination or proctoscopy is usually impossible because of pain. Examination under anaesthesia (EUA) may confirm the diagnosis, but is rarely needed.
- ■ *Treatment*: GTN ointment (0.2%) topically. Internal anal sphincterotomy is used in resistant or unresponsive cases (Jonas & Schofield 2004).

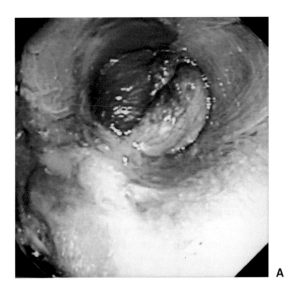

A

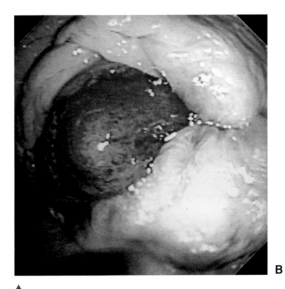

B

Fig. 9.1 A Proctoscopic view of two internal haemorrhoids. **B** Prolapsed (third degree) haemorrhoid with associated rectal mucosa prolapse (seen as surrounding pale rim of tissue). (Courtesy of Mr A. Watson and the Medical Illustration Department, Manchester Royal Infirmary, Manchester.)

Solitary rectal ulcer syndrome

This usually presents with rectal bleeding, often in constipated patients who strain excessively. The ulcer is thought to be caused by partial prolapse of the rectal mucosa with subsequent ischaemic damage and ulceration. Patients may also give a history of digitation/instrumentation. It is diagnosed at sigmoidoscopy, with biopsy to exclude other causes of ulceration (e.g. carcinoma, Crohn's disease).

■ *Treatment*: treat the underlying constipation with education, perhaps extending to biofeedback therapy, to prevent excessive straining.

Sexually transmitted disease

Most often this is gonococcal proctitis from anal intercourse. A careful history will usually suggest the diagnosis. Rectal biopsy and culture confirm the diagnosis.

Proctitis

Distal inflammatory bowel disease may present solely as rectal bleeding without accompanying diarrhoea.

9.19 Should proctoscopy/rigid sigmoidoscopy be performed routinely in primary care as part of the evaluation of patients with rectal bleeding?

Endoscopic practice, with the rest of medicine, is gradually moving towards competency-based assessment of different techniques. This kind of assessment of gastroscopists and colonoscopists, to name only two, is imminent and may be carried out in either the primary or secondary care setting. We feel that proctoscopy and rigid sigmoidoscopy should be subjected to a similar assessment process. If the healthcare practitioner has been assessed to be competent to perform a particular procedure and, crucially, is performing enough procedures every year to maintain competence, then there is no reason why these procedures should not be performed in primary care.

POLYPS

9.20 What are the different types of polyp?

Polyps may be adenomatous, with or without villous configuration, or hyperplastic. Adenomas have malignant potential (around 10% become invasive malignancy) and are more likely to become invasive with increasing size (neoplastic transformation highly unlikely at <1 cm). Such polyps need surveillance according to published guidelines (*see Ch. 12*). Hyperplastic polyps are thought to have no or minimal malignant potential and do not need colonic surveillance.

Patients with chronic inflammatory bowel disease also develop so-called 'pseudo-polyps' which are areas of normal mucosa between larger areas denuded by the inflammatory process. Of themselves, pseudo-polyps have no malignant potential. Inflammatory polyps likewise have no malignant potential.

9.21 What are the hereditary polyp syndromes?

These include familial hereditary non-polyposis colorectal cancer and familial adenomatous polyposis (*see* Q 9.7).

 PATIENT QUESTIONS

9.22 I am 25 and have noticed some bright red blood on the toilet paper. Does this need investigating?

The most likely cause by far is haemorrhoids. Any serious pathology is highly unlikely, especially in the absence of any other symptoms (e.g. weight loss, prolonged diarrhoea) or a significant family history of bowel cancer (e.g. first degree relative aged under 45). Such patients may benefit from non-urgent referral to secondary care to have their presumed haemorrhoids treated, usually in the colorectal surgical clinic.

9.23 My father had bowel cancer. What chance is there that I will too?

Lifetime risk for developing bowel cancer without any other risk factor is 1 in 30. Risk of dying from bowel cancer is 1 in 50. With one first degree relative diagnosed with bowel cancer over the age of 45, this risk increases to 1 in 16. Current guidance suggests that only those with a first degree relative diagnosed under the age of 45 (with a lifetime risk of 1 in 10, or with two first degree relatives diagnosed at any age) should be offered screening (*see* Ch. 12).

9.24 Are there any diets that would protect me from developing bowel cancer?

There is no 'protective diet' to prevent bowel cancer but increasing evidence suggests that a diet relatively low in red meat and high in fibre and fresh fruit and vegetables is beneficial in this respect.

9.25 I have diverticular disease. Should I follow a specific diet?

There is no specific diet for patients with diverticular disease. Traditionally, a high fibre diet has been recommended but there is little evidence that this strategy is effective in preventing attacks of acute diverticulitis.

9.26 How likely is diverticular disease to become cancer?

Diverticular disease does not increase the likelihood of bowel cancer.

9.27 I have colonic polyps. Will I get bowel cancer?

Only 10% of polyps turn into bowel cancer and it takes small polyps many years (perhaps as many as 15) to become cancerous. Nevertheless, it is important to remove any significant polyps, which we know reduces the risk of developing bowel cancer.

Extraintestinal manifestations of gastrointestinal tract disease

10

Diseases of the gastrointestinal tract may present with symptoms and signs relating to other systems within the body; conversely, the complications of gastrointestinal disease may also affect other systems (*Table 10.1*).

10.1 How can gastrointestinal disease affect the eyes?

Apart from icterus and anaemia, the eyes can also display the following signs in association with gastrointestinal disease:

- *Xanthelasmata* – yellowish-white plaques on the upper and lower eyelids. Seen particularly in middle-aged females with primary biliary cirrhosis. Such patients also have intense pruritus and generalised hyperpigmentation.
- *Kayser–Fleischer rings* – brown rings of copper deposited around the iris; seen in Wilson's disease. Kayser–Fleischer rings cannot be seen at the bedside; detection requires referral to ophthalmology and a slit-lamp examination.
- *Conjunctivitis, episcleritis and iritis* – all associated with inflammatory bowel disease, particularly Crohn's disease, and related to disease activity (*see Table 10.1*).

10.2 Which skin rashes are associated with gastrointestinal disease?

- *Dermatitis herpetiformis* – blistering, itchy rash on extensor surfaces, shoulders, elbows and buttocks. Over 90% have coeliac disease but less

TABLE 10.1 Extraintestinal manifestations of inflammatory bowel disease

System	Crohn's disease*	Ulcerative colitis*	Both
Skin	Aphthous ulcers[†]		Erythema nodosum[†]
			Pyoderma gangrenosum
Joints	Finger clubbing[†]		Large joint arthritis[†]
			Small joint arthritis
			Sacroiliitis
Liver	Gallstones	Primary sclerosing cholangitis and cholangiocarcinoma	Abnormal LFTs common
Renal	Stones		
Eyes			Conjunctivitis/ episcleritis/iritis[†]
Blood			Hypercoagulable state[†] in flare-up of disease

* Proctocolectomy relieves extraintestinal manifestations in ulcerative colitis, but not in Crohn's disease.
[†] Associated with disease activity.

than 5% of dermatitis herpetiformis patients have any appreciable gastrointestinal symptoms. Virtually all patients, whether coeliac or not, respond to a gluten-free diet. Occasionally dapsone is required.

■ *Erythema nodosum* – associated with active inflammatory bowel disease, particularly Crohn's disease. Painful purple–red swellings over the shins, healing without scarring. Occurs in 7% of Crohn's patients and 4% of ulcerative colitis patients. Other causes include tuberculosis, streptococcal infection, sarcoid and drugs (including the oral contraceptive pill).

■ *Pyoderma gangrenosum* – solitary purple–black tender ulcers, associated with inflammatory bowel disease (4% of ulcerative colitis patients, 1% of Crohn's), but unrelated to disease activity. Pyoderma gangrenosum often appears in patients with subclinical inflammatory bowel disease; however, treatment of the disease activity, if present, will often improve the lesion. Pyoderma gangrenosum is also associated with rheumatoid arthritis.

■ *Chronic liver disease*, particularly secondary to alcohol abuse, can lead to many skin abnormalities including spider naevi, purpura, palmar erythema, Dupuytren's contracture and abdominal striae. Cholestatic jaundice typically causes severe pruritus and skin irritation.

■ *Others* – various polyposis syndromes have associated skin pathology. These include multiple epidermoid cysts in familial adenomatous polyposis, mucocutaneous hyperpigmentation (especially lips and gums) in Peutz–Jeghers syndrome, and hyperpigmentation and nail dystrophy in Cronkhite–Canada syndrome. Some gastrointestinal malignancies have cutaneous markers, including gastric carcinoma underlying acanthosis nigricans, and deep or superficial venous thromboembolism, especially pancreatic carcinoma. The rare glucagon-secreting pancreatic tumour causes necrolytic migratory erythema (*Table 10.2*).

10.3 How does gastrointestinal disease affect the musculoskeletal system?

■ *Arthritis* – linked to inflammatory bowel disease (IBD). May be large joint (during active flare of disease), small joint 'sero-negative' or sacroiliitis (both unrelated to IBD activity).

■ *Osteoporosis* – either as a direct consequence of gastrointestinal disease (e.g. disturbance of calcium metabolism by malabsorption, secondary to coeliac or Crohn's disease) or more commonly secondary to prolonged steroid therapy, particularly for inflammatory bowel disease.

TABLE 10.2 Skin conditions and underlying gastrointestinal malignancy

	Skin manifestation	Gastrointestinal disease
Cancer/polyposis syndromes		
Gardner's	Multiple epidermoid cysts	Familial adenomatous polyposis
Muir–Torre	Sebaceous neoplasms	Proximal colonic cancer
Peutz–Jeghers	Hyperpigmentation of buccal mucosa	Hamartomas, occasionally duodenal carcinoma
Cowden's	Facial verrucous lesions	Hamartomatous polyps
Cronkhite–Canada	Hyperpigmentation, alopecia, nail dystrophy	Polyposis, malnutrition and malabsorption
Cutaneous markers of gastrointestinal malignancy		
Dermatomyositis	Psoriatic-like erythema, especially elbows and knees	25% have internal malignancy, especially gastric carcinoma
Tylosis	Hyperkeratotic palms and soles	Oesophageal carcinoma
Acanthosis nigricans	Velvety hyperplasia of axillae and neck	Gastric carcinoma
Carcinoid syndrome	Flushing	Carcinoid with liver metastases
Glucagonoma	Necrolytic migratory erythema	Pancreatic glucagonoma
Venous thrombosis	Superficial thromboses	Pancreatic carcinoma
Gastrointestinal neoplasms with skin metastases		
	Rarely occur	Periumbilical (Sister Mary Joseph's nodule) gastrointestinal carcinoma, especially gastric

10.4 What signs are seen in the nails in gastrointestinal disease?

■ *Leuconychia* (white nails) and *koilonychia* (spoon-shaped nails) are seen in profound hypoalbuminaemia and severe iron deficiency, respectively. Both are rarely seen in gastroenterology practice in the developed world.

■ *Clubbing* – may be seen in inflammatory bowel disease or alcoholic liver disease, and in coeliac disease.

10.5 How may the neurological system be linked to gastrointestinal disease?

■ Coeliac disease has a rare association with spinocerebellar degeneration.

■ There is an increased incidence of coeliac disease in epileptics.

Nutrition, obesity and diets

11.1 What is obesity?

Historically, obesity has meant too much adipose tissue (from the Latin *obesus*, fat and *esus*, consume). Modern definitions rely on the measurement of body mass index (BMI) which has been shown to correlate well with excess adiposity. Obesity is defined as a BMI of more than 30 kg/m².

11.2 How is body mass index calculated?

$$\text{BMI} = \text{weight in kg/height in metres squared (m}^2)$$

'Normal BMI' is defined from population studies and standard deviations from the norm (National Heart, Lung and Blood Institute 1998):

- Protein–energy malnutrition: mild, moderate, severe = 17–18.4, 16–16.9, <16
- Normal BMI = 18.5–24.9
- Overweight = 25–29.9
- Obese grade 1 = 30–34.9
- Obese grade 2 = 35–39.9
- Obese grade 3 = ≥40.0.

11.3 What impact does body shape have on risk from obesity?

The different body shapes are well described (apple, pear or 'V' shaped) and waist size has an independent effect on the consequences of obesity.

As can be seen from *Table 11.1*, the influence of waist size on health becomes less important as overall BMI increases (National Heart, Lung and Blood Institute 1998).

11.4 How common is obesity?

The prevalence of obesity varies geographically (*Table 11.2*).

TABLE 11.1 **Risk of metabolic complications from obesity**

BMI	Waist <40" (men) or <35" (women)	Waist >40" (men) or >35" (women)
18.5–24.9	–	Increased
25–29.9	Increased	High
30–34.9	High	Very high
35–39.9	Very high	Very high
40+	Extremely high	Extremely high

TABLE 11.2 Obesity rates: UK and US		
	UK* (%)	USA† (%)
Overweight	40	34
Obese	22	27
Combined data	62	61

* 2003 figures, Office for National Statistics.
† 1999 figures, National Health and Nutrition Examination Survey (NHANES), detailed in Flegal et al (2002).

11.5 Which drugs may cause weight gain?

These include antipsychotics, tricyclic antidepressants, monoamine oxidase inhibitors, lithium and steroids.

11.6 Which diseases are definitely linked to obesity?

Increasing BMI correlates with hypertension, diabetes and an abnormal lipid profile – all of which increase the risk of ischaemic heart disease. Obesity is also an independent risk factor for congestive cardiac failure, as well as being linked to the development of osteoarthritis and sleep apnoea syndrome (and its consequences, including right heart failure).

In females, obesity is linked to amenorrhoea and menstrual irregularity as well hirsutism. Weight gain in women increases the risk of breast cancer.

11.7 Which gastrointestinal diseases are linked to obesity?

Obesity is linked with the following gastrointestinal diseases:

- reflux oesophagitis, Barrett's oesophagus and oesophageal adenocarcinoma
- gallstones and gallbladder cancer (particularly in females)
- fatty liver – non-alcoholic fatty liver disease (NAFLD); non-alcoholic steatohepatitis (NASH)
- pancreatitis (because of gallstones, lipid abnormalities)
- colonic polyps and colonic cancer, particularly for men and particularly with increased waist to hip ratios.

11.8 What causes obesity?

Obesity, put simply, is caused by an excess of calories consumed compared with calories expended. 'To lose weight, eat less, exercise more or both.' Behind this simplistic statement is a more complex causation. Genetics certainly has a role to play in obesity but probably less than the average obese person thinks. The proportion of fast twitch and slow twitch muscle fibres (which determine efficiency of calorie burning) is partially determined by genetics but can be altered by diet and exercise.

11.9 What is the differential diagnosis of obesity?

Rare secondary causes need to be excluded. These include hypothalamic tumours such as craniopharyngioma, injury to the hypothalamic appetite centre, Cushing's disease, hypothyroidism, Prader–Willi syndrome (morbid obesity from childhood, learning difficulties, microgenitalia, short stature) and drugs (*see* Q 11.5).

11.10 Which weight-reducing diets have been shown to work?

Any dietary/exercise regime will result in weight loss if calories expended exceed calories consumed. No particular diet has been shown to be superior to another in this respect by controlled trials.

11.11 What is the drug treatment of obesity?

The drug treatment of obesity should be reserved for those with a BMI of more than 30 kg/m^2 or more than 28 kg/m^2 if other risk factors such as type 2 diabetes or hypercholesterolaemia are present.

There are two drugs currently licensed for use in the UK and they have been the subject of National Institute for Clinical Excellence (NICE) guidance (NICE 2001, BNF 2005). Orlistat (120 mg daily) is a pancreatic lipase inhibitor shown in controlled trials to reduce body weight by 2–6 kg. Important side-effects include disturbance of bowel function, including episodic incontinence, and malabsorption of fat-soluble vitamins. NICE has recommended that treatment should be continued beyond 6 months only if at least 10% weight loss has been achieved.

Fenfluramine and dexfenfluramine – amfetamines used historically – have both been withdrawn following concerns about valvular heart disease. The only licensed centrally acting appetite suppressant still licensed in the UK is sibutramine – an inhibitor of reuptake of noradrenaline and serotonin. It is not licensed for use beyond 12 months.

11.12 What is the future of drug treatment in obesity?

This is an area of active research. Leptins have been shown in early trials to achieve similar reduction in weight to orlistat (Heymsfield et al 1999).

11.13 Which surgical treatments are effective in obesity?

Obesity surgery has a high media profile. It should only be used as the last resort in the most severe, potentially life-threatening cases. Guidelines suggest it should be used as a treatment only if BMI exceeds 40 kg/m^2 (or

>35 kg/m² if severe co-morbidity is present). The correct term is bariatric surgery (from the Greek *baros* for weight).

Techniques can be divided into those that diminish the gastric reservoir and those that induce malabsorption. The two methods can be seen as complementary and are often combined as gastric bypass surgery which consists of gastric pouch formation with a jejunal loop anastomosing this pouch to the distal duodenum. Such surgery can achieve dramatic and sustained weight loss but is not without complications, including perioperative mortality of around 1–2%. Postoperative complications include dumping, constipation and vitamin B12 deficiency.

11.14 What is malnutrition?

Malnutrition is an imbalance between intake of nutrients and expenditure. It may be a generalised protein–energy malnutrition or a lack of specific nutrients.

Generalised protein–energy malnutrition is well recognised in particular crises in the developing world but is also common in hospitalised inpatients in the developed world, particularly frail, elderly patients admitted with serious physical and/or mental illness. Some studies suggest up to 50% of such patients may be malnourished. Such issues are readily explored by a dietitian's dietetic history and calorie intake assessment. Weight loss of >10% in less than 3 months and/or a BMI of less than 19 strongly suggests malnutrition.

11.15 What is enteral nutrition?

Enteral nutrition refers to nutritional support àdministered using the gut. This ranges from oral supplements through nasogastric feeding to percutaneous endoscopic gastrostomy (PEG) feeding. Enteral nutrition is always preferred to parenteral nutrition (*see Q 11.16*) because there are fewer potential complications and gut essential nutrients (e.g. glutamine) can be delivered to the gastrointestinal mucosa.

When oral intake is not possible or wholly inadequate, the patient must be tube fed. Short-term tube feeding uses a nasogastric tube. For longer term tube feeding, this is achieved by a gastrostomy tube – a tube placed through the abdominal wall endoscopically, radiologically or, less commonly, surgically (*see Q 13.11*). Patients are typically those with neurological disease (e.g. cerebrovascular accident, motor neurone disease) or head and neck cancer. In either case, the tube may be sited permanently or temporarily, allowing improvement in symptoms or treatment (radiotherapy or surgery) to take place.

If the tube is removed accidentally (usually without ill effect), it must be replaced or the track maintained using a Foley catheter or similar, within

12–24 hours at most. After this period of time, the track closes and a whole new procedure may be needed. Tubes must be replaced periodically to avoid leakage/wear. This can be done with or without endoscopy. Shorter length tubes are available for more acceptable cosmesis. PEG tubes are associated with 0.5% mortality and complications in 10%. The 30-day mortality can be as high as 30%, largely reflecting the serious underlying illness necessitating PEG insertion (Nicholson et al 2000).

11.16 What is parenteral nutrition?

Parenteral nutrition means using the vascular system to provide nutrition in cases where the gut does not function. This can be either short term (e.g. severe burns, multiple trauma, postoperatively) or long term (e.g. post bowel infarction).

Parenteral nutrition may be administered peripherally in the short term. Longer term treatment requires central venous cannulation, usually using a tunnelled or Hickman central line. Such treatment is expensive and has many potential complications (line infection/septicaemia, liver damage, metabolic bone disease) and should be reserved for situations when enteral nutrition is entirely contraindicated.

In patients on home parenteral nutrition (HPN), the annual survival rate is 80+%, with 6% of patients dying per year due to HPN-related complications (usually catheter sepsis). Median survival for such patients is around 5 years.

11.17 Which gastrointestinal diseases present with particular deficiencies?

Lack of specific nutrients may point towards a specific underlying disease state.

- *Coeliac disease* – may present with iron- or folate-deficient anaemia or metabolic bone disease secondary to vitamin D malabsorption.
- *Pernicious anaemia* – autoimmune disease characterised by vitamin B12 deficiency caused by destruction of intrinsic factor-producing cells of the stomach.
- *Chronic pancreatitis* – as well as generalised malabsorption with steatorrhoea, chronic pancreatitis may lead to specific deficiency of fat-soluble vitamins (A, D, E and K) with the potential complications of night-blindness (A), bone disease and proximal myopathy (D), cerebellar disease (E) or disordered clotting with easy bruising (K). Chronic liver cholestasis (e.g. due to primary biliary cirrhosis) can also lead to similar deficiency problems.
- *Crohn's disease* – as well as generalised malabsorption due to widespread small bowel disease or following extensive small bowel

resection, Crohn's patients tend to suffer from vitamin B12 deficiency, either due to disease in the terminal ileum or following resection of this area during a right hemicolectomy* – the commonest operation performed in Crohn's patients.

■ *Bacterial overgrowth* – this may be due to small bowel diverticulae or occur as part of the blind loop syndrome in postsurgical patients. As well as causing diarrhoea due to generalised malabsorption, such bacteria may competitively consume vitamin B12, leading to deficiency.

11.18 Which specialist diets are used in gastroenterology?

■ *Gluten-free diet* (coeliac disease) – complete avoidance of gluten reduces both symptoms and the risk of developing ulcerative jejunitis and small bowel lymphoma. The Coeliac Society (see Appendix) provides excellent advice, as do both primary and secondary care dietitians. Avoidance of wheat, barley, oats and rye is usually recommended but ongoing debate exists about how important each of these (apart from wheat) is to effective treatment. A gluten-free diet is also used for the effective management of dermatitis herpetiformis even in the absence of coeliac disease.

■ *Lactose-free diet* – hypolactasia may be temporary following a bout of acute gastroenteritis or a more permanent feature of inflammatory bowel disease or coeliac disease. All milk or milk-containing products should be avoided (substituting soya milk where possible). Butter and cheese are usually allowed.

■ *Low protein diet* – formerly used in the management of patients with hepatic encephalopathy in an attempt to reduce the protein load in the bowel. Now not commonly used as it is recognised that malnutrition is a much greater problem in such patients.

■ *Low residue diet* – infrequently used in the management of intestinal strictures (e.g. Crohn's disease). It requires a nearly complete avoidance of fibre in the diet.

■ *Elemental/polymeric diet* – the normal diet is entirely replaced by artificial liquid feeds. Elemental diets consist of free amino acids, glucose polymers and minimal fats as long-chain triglycerides. They are relatively unpalatable (sometimes requiring nasogastric feeding) and expensive. They were used initially as an effective treatment for

---

* All Crohn's disease patients must be given life-long intramuscular vitamin B12 injections following right hemicolectomy. Such patients may also experience diarrhoea postoperatively because of bile salt malabsorption (rather than due to colonic inflammation or other reason). This can often be effectively treated with a bile salt-binding agent such as colestyramine.

Crohn's disease (60% response at 6 weeks in active disease). Their use has now largely been superseded by polymeric feeds, which are better tolerated and contain whole proteins. They seem equally effective in managing such patients.

■ *Low salt diet* – indicated for fluid retention (e.g. in ascites due to liver disease). 'No salt' diets are extremely unpalatable and presently 'No added (table) salt' diets are recommended for such patients.

■ *Exclusion diet* – indicated when food intolerance seems to play a role in symptoms, especially of irritable bowel syndrome. Requires good patient motivation and enthusiastic dietetic support. The diet is initially restricted to a very small number of foods with others being slowly introduced at fortnightly intervals. If tolerated, such diets can help symptoms in up to half of affected patients; however, they are difficult to maintain.

11.19 What is anorexia nervosa?

First described in the 17th century and affecting around 0.3% of teenage girls (90% are female) and 0.02% of teenage boys, most develop the disease between puberty and age 25. Certain occupations have a higher prevalence – for example, up to 20% of ballet dancers may have anorexia.

There are four diagnostic criteria:

■ Refusal to maintain minimally normal body weight
■ Fear of becoming fat
■ Disordered body image (refusal to acknowledge low body weight)
■ Amenorrhoea.

Onset may be preceded or accompanied by an intense physical exercise regime. Between 20 and 50% of patients report a history of sexual abuse.

BMI is typically less than 17.5 kg/m^2 and 70% have lanugo hair.

Hypokalaemia is common and may indicate self-induced vomiting; if severe, this can cause ECG abnormalities. Patients may have accelerated dental erosions (from repeated vomiting), and other gastrointestinal manifestations (gut motility disturbance, liver abnormalities and pancreatitis) are relatively common.

Management is challenging and best achieved by a multidisciplinary approach including psychiatrist, physician, dietitian and family members. Nutritional support may be needed in the most severe cases and patients must be closely monitored as catastrophic changes in electrolytes may occur. Cognitive therapy can be effective in contrast to drug measures which seem to prolong the illness in some cases.

Up to 70% of patients achieve and maintain a normal body weight. On the other hand, lifetime incidence of obsessive–compulsive disorder can be as high as 25%.

11.20 What is bulimia?

First described in the 1970s, patients with bulimia nervosa are typically normal or even overweight. The illness is characterised by recurrent binge eating followed by vomiting, use of purgatives or overexercise. It is commoner than anorexia, with a lifetime prevalence in women approaching 5%, and tends to affect an older age group in their twenties.

BMI is usually normal but up to 50% of patients have parotid enlargement, and dental erosions (together with callosities on the knuckles) are common.

Combination cognitive–behavioural therapy seems the most effective treatment but antidepressants can also reduce the frequency of vomiting episodes.

Around 70% of patients cease abnormal bingeing behaviour but intermittent, infrequent relapse is common.

 PATIENT QUESTIONS

11.21 I am overweight but I don't eat much. Could it be my glands?

Rarely are patients overweight because of underlying medical illness, most commonly an underactive thyroid gland. Much more common is that you consume more energy (or calories) in food than you expend in exercise. Reducing your intake and increasing energy expenditure is the one sure way of guaranteeing weight reduction.

11.22 I want drugs and/or surgery for my weight problem. Where can I go to have this?

Drugs and surgery are reserved for those with severe obesity problems who have already failed to lose weight following a controlled diet/exercise regime. Both are only ever used as part of a comprehensive treatment plan, involving diet and exercise. Both treatments also have appreciable side-effects and, in the case of surgery, associated risk of death.

Screening and surveillance in gastroenterology

12.1 What is screening, what is surveillance?

Screening refers to the testing of the asymptomatic population to detect a subgroup that is at higher risk of either having or developing the specific condition. A screening test should be cheap, safe, accurate, readily available and acceptable. Surveillance refers to serial investigation of an identified group at higher risk of developing a disease, with the intent of detecting the condition earlier and thereby reducing mortality.

12.2 Which screening or surveillance tools are available in gastroenterology?

Several modalities are used in common practice. They include blood tests (e.g. the tumour markers carcinoembryonic antigen (CEA), CA19-9 and alphafetoprotein (AFP)), faecal occult bloods (FOBs), ultrasound scanning (usually in combination with AFP testing) and endoscopy (gastroscopy, flexible sigmoidoscopy, colonoscopy; *see Ch. 13*).

12.3 What do sensitivity, specificity and positive predictive value mean?

As a prerequisite to clinical use it is imperative that the sensitivity (i.e. how well it detects those with the disease) and the specificity (i.e. how well it detects those who do not have the disease) of the test are appreciated. In clinical practice, however, the most important aspects for the physician are the positive and negative predictive values (PPV and NPV) of the test. The PPV of a test tells the physician how likely it is that the person tested actually has the disease if the test returns positive (and NPV how likely it is that the person tested does not have the disease if the test is negative).

The PPV of a test is crucially dependent on the *specificity* and also the *prevalence* of the disease in the population studied. The PPV is defined as the 'true' positives divided by all the positive results ('true' positives plus 'false' positives).

A high PPV necessitates a denominator which is numerically similar to the numerator (i.e. it requires that the 'false' positives are few). It is therefore critically dependent on the specificity of the test. A specificity of 100% means that the test correctly identifies all those who do not have the disease (in other words, there are no people who do not have the disease who test positive, i.e. there are no 'false' positives). If specificity falls to 99%, there will be 1 false-positive test per 100 subjects screened. The importance of specificity can be illustrated in the following example. Let us say that one wishes to detect diabetes (1 in 50) in a population of 10 000 (i.e. there are 200 diabetics within this population) and the test employed has a sensitivity of 100% and a specificity of 99%. There will be 200 'true' positives and 100 'false' positives detected. This would result in a high PPV (200/200 + 100 =

67%). If, however, the specificity of the test fell to 90%, then there would be 10 false positives per 100 screened, i.e. 1000 false positives, and the PPV would fall dramatically (200/200 + 1000 = 17%). Sensitivity has less influence on the PPV. If the sensitivity fell to 90%, with a specificity of 99%, then 180 of the 200 diabetics would be identified (i.e. 180 'true' positives) and there would still be 100 'false' positives. This would result in only a tiny fall in the PPV (180/180 + 100 = 64%).

Prevalence of the disease in the population studied is also critical. Assuming a sensitivity of 100% and a specificity of 99%, if the prevalence of disease is fairly high, say diabetes (1 in 50), then if 10 000 subjects are screened, there will be 200 'true' positives detected and 100 'false' positives. This would result in a high PPV (200/200 + 100 = 67%). If, however, the prevalence of the disease in the population studied is much lower, say ulcerative colitis (1 in 1000), then with the same test attributes (100% sensitivity, 99% specificity), there will be 10 'true' positives detected out of the 10 000 screened and 100 'false' positives. This would result in a low PPV (10/10 + 100 = 9%).

It can therefore be seen that specificity needs to be very high, otherwise there will be large numbers of individuals with false-positive tests who are then subjected to further needless and potentially harmful investigations or treatments. Equally, and crucially, if the specificity is not 100%, and the less prevalent the disease in the population to which the test is applied, the lower the PPV and the less meaningful the test is to the physician in deciding whether or not that particular individual has the condition.

12.4 How useful is carcinoembryonic antigen testing?

Carcinoembryonic antigen (CEA) is the most extensively studied tumour marker. CEA is not specific for colorectal cancer (CRC) and elevations are found in patients with other gastrointestinal cancers (e.g. gastric, pancreatic and hepatic carcinomas), as well as in non-gastrointestinal tract cancers (e.g. breast and lung). It is present in low levels in normal healthy subjects, but over 98% have levels below 5 ng/ml. Levels tend to be higher in males and in smokers although almost never above 10 ng/ml.

CEA has poor sensitivity for detecting CRC (at a cut off of 5 ng/ml). In a study of 358 patients with resected CRC, preoperative elevated levels were present in only 4% of Dukes A, 25% of Dukes B and 44% of Dukes C carcinomas. Even when distant metastases were present, CEA was abnormal in only 65% of patients (Wanebo et al 1978).

The value of CEA measurement in detecting asymptomatic carcinoma (gastrointestinal and extraintestinal) in the general population is limited. In 1969, 2372 subjects aged 40 and over in Western Australia had blood taken and stored as part of a triennial health examination. Subsequent assays showed that 73 (3%) had CEA levels >5 ng/ml. Over the next 5 years (without knowledge of the CEA status), 9/73 (13%) developed 'CEA-associated tumours', compared to 25/2299 (1%) who developed 'CEA-associated tumours' with normal CEA levels. This translates into a sensitivity of 26%, a specificity of 97% and a PPV of 12%. Of the 34 'CEA-associated tumours', 7 were colorectal, and only 2/7 had CEA levels >5 ng/ml, giving a sensitivity of 29%, a specificity of 97% and a PPV of just 2.7% for the detection of CRC (Cullen et al 1976). In other words, based on a CEA >5 ng/ml, there would be 37 false positives for every one patient found to have CRC and over two-thirds of these cancers would be missed.

12.5 Is a carcinoembryonic antigen measurement any help in deciding whether a patient with abdominal symptoms needs further investigation?

One study has assessed the performance of CEA in detecting CRC in a 'high risk' population. CEA levels were performed early in the course of investigation in 97 patients with lower gastrointestinal symptoms (altered bowel habit or rectal bleeding). Malignancy was diagnosed in 38 of the 97 patients and, in 22 of these 38, the CEA level (cut off 9 ng/ml) was elevated (sensitivity 58%). In 11 of the 59 patients without malignancy, the CEA level was also raised, giving a specificity of 81% and a PPV of 66%. Every case of malignancy was, however, detected by routine investigation, with CEA measurement not adding any further diagnostic benefit (Hine et al 1978).

12.6 How useful is CA19-9 testing?

CA19-9 antigen is a sialylated form of the Lewis[a] antigen. Since 5% of the population do not express the Lewis[a] antigen, the sensitivity of CA19-9 for detecting carcinoma is limited at most to 95%. CA19-9, like CEA, is tumour associated, but not tumour specific. It is synthesised by pancreatic and biliary duct cells, and gastric, colonic and endometrial cells, but very little appears in the blood of healthy controls. At the usual cut-off value of 37 units/ml, CA19-9 has a sensitivity for pancreatic carcinoma of 80% and a specificity of 90% (Steinberg 1990). Due to the very low prevalence of pancreatic carcinoma in the asymptomatic general population, it has no role in mass screening.

In the hospital setting, the usual dilemma is distinguishing benign from malignant pancreatic disease, and in this setting the performance of CA19-9 is impressive. In a study of 250 patients with pancreatic disease (pancreatic carcinoma 99, chronic pancreatitis 121, and acute pancreatitis 30), the sensitivity was 83%, specificity 92%, PPV 87% and NPV 89% for pancreatic carcinoma, using a cut-off value of 37 units/ml. If differentiating between carcinoma and chronic pancreatitis only, the PPV rises to 94% due to the increased specificity (96%). In this study all cases of chronic pancreatitis had CA19-9 levels ≤90 units/ml except two cases with values of 120 units/ml which were subsequently found to have laryngeal and pharyngeal carcinomas (Piantino et al 1986). A further study confirms these findings with a PPV of 74% and NPV of 97% for pancreatic carcinoma using a cut-off value of 75 units/ml in differentiating between pancreatic carcinoma and benign jaundice, benign pancreatic disease, non-pancreatic abdominal pain, non-pancreatic malabsorption and renal dialysis (Steinberg et al 1986). CA19-9 levels >1000 units/ml are virtually diagnostic of pancreatic carcinoma, with specificities of >99% (Steinberg et al 1986, Pleskow et al 1989).

12.7 What is the value of alphafetoprotein testing?

Alphafetoprotein (AFP) is a normal fetal serum protein which is synthesized by fetal liver cells and yolk sac cells. It reaches peak levels by the 12th week of gestation and declines to negligible levels during the first year of life. AFP levels are elevated in a proportion of patients with hepatocellular carcinoma (HCC), and therefore efforts have been directed to find an effective screening strategy for patients at high risk of developing HCC using interval AFP ± liver ultrasound, as detection of HCC at an asymptomatic stage has been shown to improve 5- and 10-year survival figures in a study from China (Tang et al 1993; *see also Q 12.8*).

Using a cut-off value of 10.5 ng/ml, the sensitivity of AFP for detecting HCC was 80%, with a specificity of 98% and PPV of 91% in a series from King's College Hospital, London (Johnson et al 1978). There were, however, no data on the stage (size) of tumours, which is crucial since curative resection is inversely related to the size of the tumour. Generally, single HCCs of ≤5 cm are considered potentially curable surgically, and sensitivities of AFP (>20 ng/ml) for detecting this size of tumour range between 53 and 84%. In a prospective study of 363 cirrhotics with a clinical suspicion of HCC (final prevalence 40%), an AFP >20 ng/ml was 78% sensitive, 79% specific and had a PPV of 88%. Increasing the threshold to >200 ng/ml lowered sensitivity to 64%, but increased specificity to 99.5% with a corresponding increase in the PPV to 99%. AFP >500 ng/ml was considered diagnostic in this study with a sensitivity of 49%, specificity of 100% and PPV of 100% (Maringhini et al 1988). It should be noted that the prevalence of HCC in this study group was very high, and the PPV would be much less impressive if employed in more general screening studies (e.g. asymptomatic chronic hepatitis B carriers).

12.8 How does ultrasound examination compare with alphafetoprotein testing?

Ultrasound examination (USS) has been shown to be at least as sensitive and specific as AFP in the detection of HCC in at-risk populations, and therefore the two have often been used in a complementary fashion. In a large prospective study of 432 patients with chronic (non-cirrhotic) hepatitis B infection, who were screened at 3- to 6-monthly intervals with AFP and USS, eight HCCs were detected, with six first indicated by AFP measurement and two (both with AFP <20 ng/ml) by USS (Liaw et al 1986). In a more intensive, prospective study of 140 cirrhotic patients (including chronic hepatitis B infection, post blood transfusion (hepatitis C) and alcoholic aetiologies) screened by 2-monthly AFP and 3-monthly linear array USS, 40 HCCs were detected over a mean follow-up of 41 months, with 33 initiated by USS findings in the first instance and 5 by elevated AFP levels. Furthermore, in 25 (62.5%) the tumour was $\leq$2 cm and the overall 3-year survival was 41% (Oka et al 1990).

Although serial AFP measurement and USS scanning are able to detect small HCCs, there is no definitive evidence that such a strategy is beneficial since there are no randomised controlled trials of screening or surveillance for HCC. However, a large series from China, spanning a 30-year period comparing asymptomatic HCC (detected by screening) versus symptomatic presentation, showed smaller tumour size, a greater proportion of small (<5 cm) HCCs, higher resectability rate (80% versus 47%), and higher 5-year (50.7% versus 20.6%) and 10-year (35.6% versus 15.9%) survival figures for the asymptomatic screened HCC group, suggesting that detection in the earlier asymptomatic phase leads to improved outcome (Tang et al 1993).

SCREENING FOR COLORECTAL CARCINOMA

Colorectal cancer (CRC) is the second most common cancer in the West. Preventative strategies can be defined as either primary or secondary.

Primary prevention involves identifying genetic, biological or environmental factors associated with the development of CRC and modifying or altering them. Epidemiological studies suggest that increased intake of fibre, fruit and cruciferous vegetables, and decreased fat intake, reduce CRC mortality, and that aspirin may also confer a beneficial effect. Randomised controlled trials, however, are necessary before such data are confirmed.

Secondary prevention depends upon identifying preneoplastic lesions or early cancers and removing them to reduce mortality from CRC, since survival improves with diagnosis at an earlier stage.

There are four potential screening tests for polyps and carcinomas: faecal occult blood testing, flexible sigmoidoscopy, barium enema and colonoscopy (*see Ch. 13*). For high risk groups (*see Q 12.18*), colonoscopic surveillance is the test of choice. Approximately 80% of all CRCs, however, are sporadic, occurring in individuals who do not have any particularly increased risk of developing the condition. The challenge is how best to detect those individuals who are going to develop a sporadic CRC, i.e. how best to detect early preneoplastic lesions (polyps). Colonoscopy is the most accurate method, but the resource implications would be enormous, and inevitably a small number of perforations would occur in patients with normal colons (risk approximately 1 in 1000).

The strongest evidence for screening individuals at 'average' risk for developing CRC is faecal occult blood testing.

12.9 What is faecal occult blood testing?

The faecal occult blood test (FOBT) comprises a piece of paper impregnated with guaiac. Guaiac is an organic compound which changes colour when oxidised by peroxidases or the pseudoperoxidase activity of haemoglobin. Examples of guaiac-based FOBTs are Haemoccult II and the more sensitive but less specific Haemoccult II Sensa. HemeSelect is an immunochemical test which tests specifically for human haemoglobin; it is not as sensitive as Haemoccult II Sensa, but is more specific.

It is important to remember that bleeding from the upper gastrointestinal tract (erosive oesophagitis, gastric carcinoma, vascular ectasia, etc.) may also cause a positive FOBT, and some studies have found an equal or even greater proportion of upper gastrointestinal sites than lower sites.

12.10 What causes a false-positive faecal occult blood test?

False-positive FOBTs lead to unnecessary investigation (colonoscopy) and occasional morbidity (perforation), and attempts to reduce their occurrence (i.e. increase the specificity of the test) should be made. Rare red meat, peroxidase-containing vegetables and fruits (e.g. broccoli, turnip, cauliflower, radish, cantaloupe melon), aspirin and non-steroidal anti-inflammatory drugs may all result in false-positive tests. All of the above should be avoided for 3 days before and during the test.

12.11 What causes a false-negative faecal occult blood test?

False-negative FOBTs are inevitable because polyps and carcinomas do not bleed all of the time. Right-sided colonic carcinomas tend to bleed much more than left-sided carcinomas and therefore tend to produce fewer false-negative results.

Vitamin C ingestion may cause false-negative FOBTs.

12.12   What does a positive faecal occult blood test mean?

A large study comparing four different FOBT regimes in over 8000 healthy subjects (aged ≥50) found that the PPV of a positive test for carcinoma was (%[95% CI]): Haemoccult II = 6.6 [3.7–11.2]; Haemoccult II Sensa = 2.5 [1.7–3.7]; HemeSelect = 5.0 [3.2–7.6]; combined Haemoccult II Sensa and HemeSelect (to confirm true positivity of Haemoccult II Sensa) = 9.0 [5.8–13.6] (Allison et al 1996). In other words, there is approximately a 2–6% chance of an individual positive FOBT actually reflecting the presence of CRC.

The PPV of a positive test for polyps ≥1 cm was: Haemoccult II = 16.7 [11.9–22.8]; Haemoccult II Sensa = 6.7 [5.3–8.4]; HemeSelect = 15.5 [12.3–19.3]; combined Haemoccult II Sensa and HemeSelect = 21.9 [16.9–27.9]. In other words, there is approximately a 6–17% chance of an individual positive FOBT actually reflecting the presence of a large (>1 cm) polyp.

The PPV for colorectal neoplasia (carcinoma or polyp ≥1 cm) was: Haemoccult II = 23.2 [17.7–29.9]; Haemoccult II Sensa = 9.2 [7.6–11.2]; HemeSelect = 20.5 [16.8–24.6]; combined Haemoccult II Sensa and HemeSelect = 30.9 [25.1–37.3]. In other words, there is approximately a 9–23% chance of an individual positive FOBT actually reflecting the presence of either a carcinoma or large polyp (Allison et al 1996).

12.13   Should I perform faecal occult blood testing in the outpatient setting to guide further investigation?

No. Patients who have lower gastrointestinal tract symptoms should be investigated conventionally. If the patient has a recent change in bowel habit, they should have the appropriate investigation (e.g. colonoscopy or barium enema). A negative FOBT in this setting may be a 'false negative' and cause false reassurance. Equally, a young person with classic symptoms of irritable bowel syndrome in whom an FOBT is performed and is positive, may well be subjected to invasive procedures inappropriately if the test is a 'false positive'. The only evidence for the use of faecal occult blood testing is in the context of a screening programme, and in such a setting it is not performed as a one-off test, but as a periodic examination.

12.14   Does the screening of healthy populations by faecal occult blood testing reduce mortality from colorectal carcinoma?

There have been several large randomised trials of faecal occult blood testing offered to the general population aged 45–50 years and older. The Nottingham trial (Hardcastle et al 1996) is the largest, involving over 150 000 subjects, and showed a 15% reduction in CRC mortality. The

Minnesota trial (Mandel et al 1993), involving 46 000 subjects, showed a 33% reduction in CRC mortality with an annual faecal occult blood screening programme, although this may in part be due to the high colonoscopy rate (38%) in this study. A meta-analysis of the randomised trials from Nottingham, Minnesota, Funen and Goteburg, published in the Cochrane Library, shows an overall significant reduction in CRC mortality using FOBT of 16% (95% CI, 8–23%) (Towler et al 1998).

12.15 What are the problems of mass faecal occult blood screening?

A screening test should be cheap, safe, sensitive, specific, acceptable and cost-effective. Faecal occult blood testing is certainly cheap and safe. Since colorectal carcinomas and polyps bleed intermittently and to variable degrees, three consecutive stools should be tested. The sensitivity of a single FOBT for detecting colorectal carcinoma is only 50–60% (i.e. there will be 40–50% false-negative tests). If three stool samples are taken, the overall sensitivity of the test rises to 70%.

As the caecum and ascending colon are wider bore sections of the colon, tumours are able to reach a larger size before becoming symptomatic, and because of their size will tend to bleed more. It is for this reason that faecal occult blood testing is most sensitive for detecting right-sided tumours (>80% sensitivity) (Macrae & St John 1982).

One of the major problems is the acceptability of the test. In the Nottingham UK study population (Hardcastle et al 1996), only 50% of those offered screening were compliant.

12.16 Is flexible sigmoidoscopy useful for screening?

The rationale for this strategy is that 65–75% of adenomatous polyps and 40–65% of colorectal cancers are within reach of a 60 cm flexible endoscope. A positive examination requires colonoscopy as the presence of distal adenomas increases the risk of more proximal lesions. More recent data suggest, however, that 40–50% of proximal cancers have no associated distal polyps (Gondal et al 2003).

No endoscopic study has shown reduced incidence of disease or reduction of mortality in a large randomised population-based study. Recent case-control studies, however, showed a 60% reduction in mortality from distal colonic and rectal carcinomas in individuals who had undergone a sigmoidoscopy (Selby et al 1992, Muller & Sonnenberg 1995).

12.17 Is colonoscopy useful for screening?

This is the 'gold standard' for assessment of the colon and allows polypectomy, but is expensive and needs skilled operators who are in short supply. It is also associated with not inconsiderable risk. In the National Polyp Study from the USA, 1418 individuals who had polyps removed at colonoscopy underwent periodic colonoscopy over an average 5.9-year follow-up period. The incidence rate of CRC was compared to three reference groups, and colonoscopic surveillance with polypectomy was shown to lower the expected incidence of CRC by 76–90% (Winawer et al 1993). Its utility as a screening tool in an asymptomatic, low risk population is untested.

12.18 What are the pros and cons on screening for colorectal cancer?

Screening asymptomatic low risk populations for colorectal cancer remains controversial (Atkin & Northover 2003, Macafee & Scholefield 2003). There is general agreement that such screening should be performed but debate remains around the exact modality. A national screening programme will start in the UK in 2006, focusing on those aged over 55, using faecal occult blood testing as an initial screen, with colonoscopy offered to those with positive tests.

In the USA, the American Cancer Society guidelines (Byers et al 1997) recommend that all individuals ≥50 years old, who are at 'average' risk (i.e. no previous polyps or CRC, no first degree relative with polyps or CRC <60 years old, and not more than two first degree relatives of any age with polyps or CRC) should be offered either faecal occult blood testing plus flexible sigmoidoscopy, or total colonic examination with colonoscopy or double contrast barium enema. If faecal occult blood testing plus flexible sigmoidoscopy is used, faecal occult blood testing should be annually and flexible sigmoidoscopy 5 yearly. If total colonic examination is used, colonoscopy is recommended 10 yearly or barium enema 5–10 yearly. Screening should stop when significant co-morbidity exists.

Although 70–80% of CRCs occur in low or 'average' risk individuals, 20–30% occur in individuals who are at increased risk either because of a significant family history of CRC or because they have an inherited condition with high risk of CRC development (e.g. familial adenomatous polyposis, hereditary non-polyposis colorectal cancer). Individuals in these higher risk groups need surveillance.

12.19 Who needs surveillance for bowel cancer?

There are a number of disease groups (*Box 12.1*) or family history groups (*Table 12.1*) for which surveillance for bowel cancer is currently indicated. This subject has been recently dealt with in a comprehensive British Society of Gastroenterology/Association of Coloproctology document (Cairns & Scholefield 2002).

One affected first degree relative over the age of 45 does not confer a risk of colorectal cancer thought to justify screening (over and above that which is offered to the general population).

> **BOX 12.1 Surveillance for bowel cancer for patients in disease groups**
>
> ▦ *Colorectal cancer*: colonoscopy within 6 months of resection and then 5 yearly until aged 70
> ▦ *Colorectal polyps*: hyperplastic polyps – no surveillance; adenomatous polyps – colonoscopic follow-up, with frequency dependent on number and type of polyps
> ▦ *Inflammatory bowel disease*: colonoscopy 8–10 years after onset of symptoms in pan-colitis, 15–20 years after left-sided colitis; colonoscopy 3 yearly in second decade (i.e. 10–20 years from onset), 2 yearly in third decade (i.e. 20–30 years from onset) and annually thereafter (i.e. >30 years from onset)
> ▦ *Inflammatory bowel disease + sclerosing cholangitis*: annual colonoscopy at diagnosis of sclerosing cholangitis
> ▦ *Ureterosigmoidoscopy*: flexible sigmoidoscopy 10 years after surgery and then annually
> ▦ *Acromegaly*: colonoscopy at 40 years and then 5 yearly

SCREENING AND SURVEILLANCE FOR OTHER TYPES OF CANCER

12.20 Who needs screening for oesophageal cancer?

There is no evidence that population screening for oesophageal cancer is justified.

12.21 Who needs surveillance for oesophageal cancer?

Patients with Barrett's oesophagus (metaplastic change of squamous to columnar epithelium in the lower oesophagus; *see* Q 2.36) are often offered regular endoscopic surveillance. There is certainly a recognised metaplasia–dysplasia–carcinoma sequence associated with Barrett's, but the absolute risk remains low. Autopsy studies show that for every diagnosed Barrett's, another 20 remain undiagnosed and cause no appreciable problem (Cameron et al 1995). The vast majority of patients with Barrett's don't die of oesophageal cancer and estimates of risk vary from 1 in 50 patient years to more than 1 in 400 patient years.

Most patients who are discovered to have developed a cancer within a Barrett's segment do so at index or first endoscopy. There are some data that patients who have cancer diagnosed as part of a surveillance programme have earlier stage disease and therefore better survival than those diagnosed outside such programmes (Wright et al 1996) but studies are small and conflicting.

TABLE 12.1 Surveillance for bowel cancer for patients in family history groups

Family group	Lifetime risk of CRC	Screening procedure	Age at initial screen	Screening procedure and interval
Familial adenomatous polyposis	100%	Genetic testing, flexible sigmoidoscopy and OGD	Puberty	Prophylactic colectomy age 16–20; 3-yearly OGD from age 30
Juvenile polyposis (JP) and Peutz–Jeghers syndrome (PJS)	JP 10–38% PJS 10–20%	Genetic testing, colonoscopy and OGD	Puberty	JP 1–2 yearly colonoscopy from age 15–18; OGD 1–2 yearly from age 25 PJS 3-yearly colonoscopy or flexible sigmoidoscopy + barium enema; 3-yearly OGD from age 25
Hereditary non-polyposis colorectal cancer (HNPCC) *	80%	Colonoscopy ± OGD	Age 25 or 5 years before youngest familial cancer, whichever is earliest OGD 50 years or 5 years before youngest gastric cancer in family	2-yearly colonoscopy and OGD
Two FDRs with CRC[†]	1 in 6 lifetime risk of dying from CRC	Colonoscopy	35–40 years	If initial colonoscopy clear, repeat at age 55
One FDR with CRC <45 years[†]	1 in 10 lifetime risk of dying from CRC	Colonoscopy	35–40 years	If initial colonoscopy clear, repeat at age 55

Adapted from Cairns & Scholefield (2002).

CRC, colorectal cancer; FDR, first degree relative; OGD, gastroscopy.

* HNPCC is defined as 3 or more family members affected by colorectal cancer, or ≥2 with CRC and one with endometrial cancer in ≥2 generations; one affected member must be aged ≤50 at diagnosis, and one of the relatives must be a first degree relative of the other two.

[†] The lifetime risk of dying from CRC in the general population is 1:50, and reduces to 1:17 if any family member is affected. Individuals with two FDRs or one FDR <45, although having a relative risk of approximately fivefold for developing CRC compared to the general population, still have a low absolute risk. It has been estimated that such individuals have a 1:1660 chance of a cancer being found aged 30–39, and that there is a 1:3618 chance that colonoscopy will prevent death from CRC. At the age of 55 however, the chance of finding a cancer falls to 1:181, and there is a 1:213 chance that colonoscopy will prevent death from CRC.

There are no randomised controlled trials comparing surveillance against non-surveillance strategies, but certain features of the Barrett's segment do confer additional risk – for example, long segment more than 8 cm, ulcer within the segment (van den Burgh et al 1996) – and perhaps it is at these patients that surveillance should be directed. Each patient should be advised not only of the small overall risk of developing cancer but also of the risks and discomfort associated with endoscopy.

Surveillance interval should be 2–3 yearly, but more frequently if biopsies reveal low grade dysplasia. Surveillance should probably cease when the patient's co-morbidity reaches a level whereby they would not survive an oesophagectomy (*see also* Q 2.40).

12.22 Who needs screening for hepatocellular carcinoma?

Recent British Society of Gastroenterology guidelines (Ryder 2003) have addressed this issue. It is recommended that all patients with cirrhosis due to hepatitis B and C, haemochromatosis, males with alcoholic cirrhosis abstinent from alcohol and males with cirrhosis due to primary biliary cirrhosis should be offered surveillance. These recommendations are based on the risk in each disease group for either sex. Surveillance should take the form of 6-monthly ultrasound scans and 6-monthly alphafetoprotein estimations, the aim being to detect small and therefore resectable tumours.

 PATIENT QUESTIONS

12.23 I am 37 years old, and my father died of bowel cancer at the age of 62. I am worried that I may have inherited his genes and would like a camera examination of my bowel.

The lifetime risk of developing bowel cancer is approximately 1 in 30, and there is a 1 in 50 chance that an individual in the general population will die from bowel cancer. The fact that there is a history of bowel cancer in your family slightly increases your risk of developing and subsequently dying of bowel cancer (1 in 17 lifetime risk) compared to the general population. Your absolute risk of having bowel cancer at your age is extremely low, and one needs to balance the risk of a colonoscopy, which has a complication rate of 1 in 300, against the extremely tiny chance of any significant pathology being found. In your situation the risks almost certainly outweigh the benefits.

In the future there will be a national screening programme looking, for example, for the presence of blood in the stool (faecal occult blood testing). Such a safe, non-invasive test may allow higher risk individuals to be selected for a colonoscopy. Alternatively, it may be that a single one-off camera examination is offered to all individuals at the age of 50–55, when the incidence of colorectal carcinoma and polyps begins to rise.

12.24 I am 33 years old and am worried because there is a lot of cancer in my family. My mother developed cancer of the uterus at the age of 40 and my maternal aunt was diagnosed with bowel cancer at the age of 48. Both of my grandfathers had bowel cancer. Do I need to be investigated?

The most important thing is that you are referred to a clinical geneticist. You do have a strong history of cancer in your family, but it is important to obtain a detailed family history to decide if you have a hereditary condition which might increase your risk of developing bowel and other cancers. The geneticist will be able to determine your risk and suggest if and how often you might need investigations (or surveillance). It is also important because, if you do have one of the rare inherited conditions predisposing you to certain cancers, this would have implications for other members of your family, including offspring.

Investigations in gastroenterology

13

13.1 What is proctoscopy?

Internal haemorrhoids cannot be palpated by an examining finger and require proctoscopy for diagnosis. A short, clear, hollow plastic tube with introducer and light source is introduced into the anal canal and distal rectum, and then slowly withdrawn, allowing visualisation of haemorrhoids (which bulge into the lumen of the tube).

13.2 What is rigid sigmoidoscopy?

A rigid hollow tube used to inspect the rectum. It may be inserted up to 25 cm. It allows inspection and biopsy of the mucosa. It is useful in confirming or refuting a flare-up of colitis. It should be used to complement a barium enema (*see* Q 13.5) since the barium is introduced via a rectal tube and therefore this region is not readily seen.

The risk of bowel perforation is extremely low, ranging between 1 in 5000 and 1 in 50 000.

13.3 What is flexible sigmoidoscopy?

A flexible video camera which may be inserted up to 60 cm beyond the anus. It is possible to inspect the colon as far as the splenic flexure or distal transverse colon (although with bowel redundancy and looping, the tip of the camera may still reside in the sigmoid colon despite 60 cm of scope inserted). It is often used to investigate bright red rectal bleeding in the younger age group since this presentation would indicate a distal origin. It may also be used to inspect and biopsy the mucosa in patients with distal colitis, acute or chronic diarrhoea (although total bowel imaging is preferable with the latter) or as a complement to a barium enema (*see* Q 13.5).

The risk of perforation is approximately 1 in 40 000.

13.4 What is colonoscopy?

A flexible video camera which allows inspection and biopsy of the whole colon and terminal ileum. It also allows hot biopsy (simultaneous biopsy and heat destruction of small polyps <5 mm), polypectomy and argon beam coagulation of angiodysplastic lesions. It is employed for assessment of bowel symptoms, screening and surveillance (e.g. for cancer in patients with inflammatory bowel disease).

Colonoscopy is the most accurate method of inspecting the colon. It has a sensitivity of approximately 95% for detecting colorectal carcinoma (compared to approximately 83% for a barium enema) (Rex et al 1997a) and, as mentioned, allows therapeutic procedures (*Fig. 13.1*).

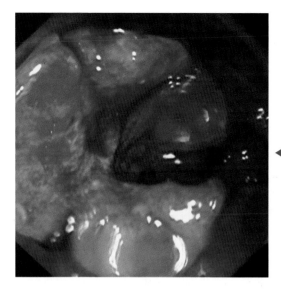

◀ **Fig. 13.1**
Colonoscopic
view of colorectal
carcinoma.
(Courtesy of
Dr Stuart Riley,
Sheffield
Teaching
Hospitals NHS
Trust, Sheffield.)

Unfortunately, it is not always technically possible to reach the caecum. A recent large survey in the UK showed that the caecal completion rate was only 77% and this fell to 57% if the criteria included either ileal intubation or positive identification of the ileocaecal valve (Bowles et al 2004). Currently there is a concerted effort to train specialist registrars in endoscopic skills, with the goal of a 90% caecal completion rate as an acceptable standard.

Colonoscopy usually requires sedation with a benzodiazepine (e.g. midazolam) with or without a small dose of an opiate.

Risks of colonoscopy include:

- ■ major complication rate: 1 in 250 (0.4%)
- ■ perforation rate: diagnostic = 1 in 1000 (0.1%); therapeutic (polypectomy etc.) = 1 in 500 (0.2%)
- ■ bleeding rate (requiring treatment/admission) = 1 in 500 (0.2%).

13.5 What is a barium enema?

Double contrast (i.e. barium and air) barium enema (DCBE) is widely used to image the colon. It is relatively cheap (compared to colonoscopy), does not require sedation and is usually complete (i.e. reaches the caecum, and often refluxes into the terminal ileum; *Fig. 13.2*). It is, however, a diagnostic test only, and involves exposure to x-rays and is less accurate than colonoscopy.

Barium enema has a lower sensitivity for detecting colorectal carcinoma (83%), with the lowest sensitivities in the sigmoid and ascending colons (around 75%). Perhaps not surprisingly, the disparity in the accuracy of barium enema and colonoscopy is greatest for the detection of polyps, particularly those less than 1 cm.

Using colonoscopy as the gold standard, barium enema has a sensitivity of only 35% for the detection of all polyps (Winawer et al 2000).

Colonoscopy also misses polyps. In a back-to-back study in which 183 patients had their colons examined by an expert colonoscopist and all polyps identified were removed, an immediate repeat colonoscopy the same day revealed that 24% of the total polyps had been missed by the first examination (Rex et al 1997b).

Barium enema should be combined with either a rigid sigmoidoscopy (since insertion of the rectal tube for administration of the barium enema renders this area 'blind') or preferably a flexible sigmoidoscopy (which allows biopsy of the mucosa, as well as visualisation of the sigmoid colon, which can be a difficult area to exclude pathology on barium radiology).

The perforation rate is negligible (1 in 25 000).

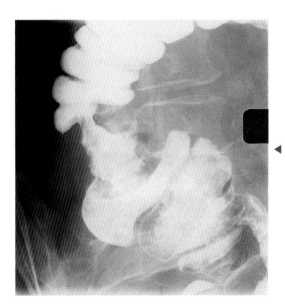

◀ Fig. 13.2 Typical 'apple-core' stricture in the ascending colon as seen on barium enema. (Courtesy of Drs C. Clout and D.J. Moore, Sheffield Teaching Hospitals NHS Trust, Sheffield.)

13.6 What is virtual colonoscopy/colonography/computed tomographic colonography?

Computed tomographic (CT) colonography is a promising new technique which involves reconstructing a three-dimensional image of the colon from two-dimensional CT slices through the abdomen (*Fig. 13.3*). It involves traditional bowel preparation and insufflation of the colon before acquisition of the CT slices.

It is attractive because it is relatively non-invasive and there is virtually no risk of perforation; it does, however, result in radiation burden. It is observer dependent, but seems to have comparable sensitivity to DCBE examination, with a sensitivity for detecting polyps ≥1 cm of approximately 50% in a low prevalence setting. In an intermediate prevalence setting it has been shown to have a sensitivity of 90% for detecting lesions ≥1 cm in size (Johnson et al 2003, Pineau et al 2003, Rex 2003). It is, however, much more costly than a barium enema.

13.7 What is oesophagogastroduodenoscopy (OGD, gastroscopy)?

This is a widely used investigation with approximately 1% of the UK population having a gastroscopy per annum. It allows diagnostic visualisation of the oesophagus, stomach and duodenum as well as biopsy (including duodenal biopsies for the diagnosis of coeliac disease).

Gastroscopy may be performed with topical throat spray anaesthesia alone (up to 50% of procedures), or with intravenous benzodiazepines.

The risks of gastroscopy include:

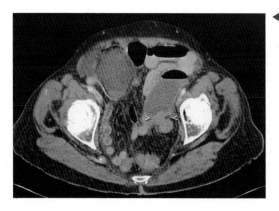

◀ **Fig. 13.3** Computed tomography scan of a sigmoid colon tumour causing large bowel obstruction. The tumour lies between the arrowheads. (Courtesy of Dr C. Clout, Sheffield Teaching Hospitals NHS Trust, Sheffield.)

■ perforation rate: 1 in 1000–3333 (0.1–0.03%), rising to 1 in 90 (1.1%) for dilatation of benign strictures and 1 in 15 (6.4%) for dilatation of malignant strictures

■ mortality: 1 in 10 000 (0.01%).

13.8 What is endoscopic retrograde cholangiopancreatography?

Endoscopic retrograde cholangiopancreatography (ERCP) is a side-viewing duodenoscope which allows visualisation and cannulation of the ampulla of Vater. Dye may then be selectively injected into the common bile duct and biliary tree or the pancreatic duct. It allows biopsies or brushings of strictures (e.g. cholangiocarcinomas, pancreatic carcinomas) and removal of common bile duct stones. It requires moderately heavy sedation with a combination of benzodiazepines and opiates.

Benefits of this technique need to be carefully balanced against risks which are considerable, for example:

■ pancreatitis (usually mild and self-limiting) occurs in approximately 5%

■ perforation of the duodenum or bleeding (after sphincterotomy) is approximately 1%

■ mortality from the procedure is approximately 1 in 1000.

13.9 What is magnetic resonance cholangiopancreatography?

Magnetic resonance cholangiopancreatography (MRCP) is a relatively recently introduced technique of imaging the pancreatic and common bile ducts using magnetic resonance. It has the huge advantage of being non-invasive (therefore risk-free), and should improve selection of patients who need ERCP, avoiding unnecessary exposure to the risks of this procedure. Consequently, the number of diagnostic ERCPs is decreasing rapidly. MRCP is in its relative infancy, but the technique and resolution are improving fast.

13.10 What is endoscopic ultrasound?

Endoscopic ultrasound (EUS) is essentially a gastroscope with a small ultrasound probe on the end. It is performed as a day-case procedure (like gastroscopy or colonoscopy) and requires light sedation.

EUS allows local ultrasound imaging and is particularly useful in staging oesophagogastric carcinomas. It is used as a complementary procedure with CT scanning. It may also be used to visualise the pancreaticobiliary system.

The earlier systems were radial scopes (giving diagnostic imaging in a transverse plane to the shaft of the scope). Linear systems now allow biopsy of EUS-targeted lesions.

The risks of the diagnostic (radial) procedure are likely to be similar to gastroscopy.

13.11 What is a percutaneous endoscopic gastrostomy tube?

This is a feeding tube inserted through the anterior abdominal wall into the stomach to allow enteral nutrition when oral intake or the swallowing mechanism is impaired. The vast majority are inserted endoscopically.

The main indication for percutaneous endoscopic gastrostomy (PEG) feeding is impaired swallowing following a cerebrovascular accident (CVA). PEG feeding tubes are often inserted prior to head and neck cancer surgery in anticipation of a prolonged period when oral intake is not possible.

Risks of PEG tube insertion include:

- minor complication rate (wound infection/excoriation) of 6–10%
- major complication rate (peritonitis, severe haemorrhage) of 2–3%
- mortality from the procedure itself of approximately 1%
- 30-day mortality rate following PEG insertion post CVA of approximately 25% (largely due to the underlying condition)
- mortality of 50% in severely demented patients who have feeding tubes inserted because of food refusal/malnutrition. This is a reflection of the end-stage of the disease, and for this reason the authors believe that PEG feeding cannot be considered beneficial for the patient and is contraindicated.

13.12 What is a barium swallow?

This is a largely outdated method of investigating the luminal upper gastrointestinal tract by radiographic examination of a patient swallowing radio-opaque liquid – specifically to examine the oesophagus and upper stomach only. It is performed unsedated in the x-ray department. It is sometimes used first line (in preference to gastroscopy) in those with dysphagia, although there is little evidence to support this approach.

Barium swallow is, however, useful in those who are intolerant of gastroscopy, have complex dysphagia problems (when a bread barium swallow may be used) or as part of the assessment of upper gastrointestinal malignancy, especially in those with apparent obstruction.

13.13 What is a barium meal?

This is similar to a barium swallow but also examines distal stomach and proximal duodenum. It was formerly the only way to diagnose duodenal ulcer preoperatively. It is now seldom used.

13.14 What is a small bowel enema/barium meal and follow-through?

This is a technique to assess the small bowel, performed in the x-ray department, unsedated.

A small bowel enema involves nasojejunal intubation and passage of contrast into the small bowel. Some patients find this uncomfortable. A barium meal and follow-through involves swallowing barium, as for a standard meal, but then the barium is followed throughout the small bowel until it reaches the terminal ileum. Each has theoretical advantages but test selection usually depends on radiologist and patient preference. It is good for detecting gross anatomical change (e.g. malrotation, Crohn's strictures, diverticulae), but is less good at detecting subtle mucosal abnormality.

13.15 What is capsule endoscopy?

This technique is now becoming widely available. It is used only when other investigations (usually including gastroscopy, colonoscopy, enteroscopy, CT scan and barium radiology) have failed to elucidate a problem. It is not used as a first line investigation in preference to these other tests, despite patient preferences.

Capsule endoscopy is useful for the investigation of obscure gastrointestinal bleeding and/or anaemia, particularly if the small bowel is the suspected source. However, it is contraindicated in suspected small bowel obstruction (may impact).

■ *Advantages* – it is relatively non-invasive, reaches the parts of the small bowel that endoscopy does not, provides good quality images of mucosal abnormalities, is popular with patients and is an attractive new technology (*Fig. 13.4*).
■ *Disadvantages* – it is diagnostic only (no biopsy or other endoscopic therapy available) and there is poor anatomical localisation with current models. In addition, it is expensive and it can be difficult to obtain funding.

13.16 What is a (radiolabelled) white cell scan?

This is used in gastroenterology for the diagnosis of inflammatory bowel disease, and for assessing activity/extent.

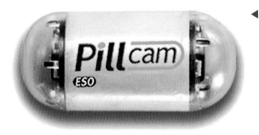

Fig. 13.4 The recently introduced capsule endoscope or 'Pill-Cam'. The size of a large tablet, it has a small but growing role in the investigation of patients with gastrointestinal symptoms. (Courtesy of Given Imaging.)

It is an outpatient test where the patient's own white cells are harvested by venepuncture and attached to a radiolabel. The radiolabelled white cells are then re-injected into the patient and migrate to the inflamed area. A gamma camera then 'photographs' the distribution of the white cells in the bowel.

13.17 What is a SeHCAT test (^{75}Se-labelled homocholic acid conjugated with taurine)?

This is a radiolabelled test of bile salt malabsorption. It involves the oral administration of labelled synthetic bile acid followed by quantitative assessment of bile acid at days 0 (100%) and 7. Normally there should be over 15% of synthetic bile salt retained (due to the enterohepatic circulation) on day 7. Bile salt malabsorption may be idiopathic, occur after cholecystectomy or may be secondary to disease or resection of the terminal ileum.

13.18 What is a glucose hydrogen breath test?

This is a test for small bowel bacterial overgrowth. It is performed fasting and having avoided poorly absorbed carbohydrates for the preceding 24 hours. It involves drinking a glucose solution, and then providing serial breath exhalations for about 2 hours. Glucose is normally rapidly absorbed in the upper small bowel and hence never comes into contact with bacteria (the small bowel is usually relatively sterile). If bacteria have populated the small bowel, they metabolise the glucose to hydrogen, which is then absorbed into the blood stream and excreted via the lungs. The test is only about 70% sensitive, since some bacteria are not hydrogen producers. The same principles apply to the lactose hydrogen breath test (*see Q 13.19*) and ^{14}C-labelled glycocholate and glycine breath tests.

13.19 What is a lactose hydrogen breath test?

This is used to diagnose lactose intolerance. Lactose is a disaccharide (glucose + galactose). Disaccharides cannot be absorbed and need to be broken down into their monosaccharide units by lactase to enable absorption. Lactose is normally broken down and absorbed in the upper gastrointestinal tract. However, in lactase deficiency, lactose cannot be broken down and enters the colon where it is fermented by bacteria with release of hydrogen, which is exhaled in the breath.

The test consists of ingestion of a standard lactose load after an overnight fast followed by serial measurement of breath hydrogen at regular intervals.

13.20 What are pancreolauryl/faecal elastase-1/PABA tests?

These are tests of pancreatic exocrine function.

■ The pancreolauryl test involves oral ingestion of fluorescein dilaurate, which is broken down by pancreatic exocrine secretions, releasing the fluorescein dye which can be measured spectrophometrically in a urine collection. The test involves a 24-hour urine collection (as an outpatient) and is only positive if more than 90% of pancreatic exocrine function is lost.

■ Faecal elastase is the faecal measurement of pancreatically produced elastase in a single faeces sample. It is more sensitive and easier to perform.

■ A PABA test involves ingestion of a non-absorbable compound which is split by pancreatic enzymes. One of the products is absorbable and subsequently detectable in a urine collection.

13.21 What is oesophageal pH and manometry?

Oesophageal manometry measures the pressure/peristalsis in the oesophageal lumen via a small catheter placed nasally. It is used to diagnose achalasia and other oesophageal motility disorders.

24-hour pH monitoring is the measurement of oesophageal pH over a 24-hour period, again using a nasally inserted catheter, and a solid-state portable recorder, like a personal stereo, which the patient takes home and brings back the following day for analysis. It is normal to have a small amount of acid reflux into the oesophagus, but this is usually rapidly cleared by oesophageal peristalsis. A pH <4 for more than 4% of the 24-hour recording period is regarded as abnormal.

13.22 What is anal manometry?

This is used to assess anal sphincter function in those with defaecatory symptoms or incontinence. It involves inserting a small tube into the rectum with a small balloon which is inflated. Sensory pressures are measured (e.g. the point at which the patient is aware of the balloon presence is recorded), as well as squeeze pressures.

13.23 What is a defaecating proctogram?

This is a radiological test performed in specialist centres only, for the evaluation of defaecatory symptoms. It involves the recording in real time of a patient defaecating a previously administered enema containing contrast in a specially designed toilet cubicle.

It is useful in diagnosing obstructive defaecatory disorders (e.g. rectoceles).

13.24 What are the different tests available for detecting the presence of *Helicobacter pylori*?

The various tests utilised in the detection of *Helicobacter pylori* are outlined in *Table 13.1*.

TABLE 13.1 Tests for the detection of *Helicobacter pylori*

Test	Description	Comments
Serology	Blood test	Sensitive (80%), cheap, rapid, but remains positive for months after successful eradication
Campylobacter-like organism (CLO) test	Gastric antral biopsy at endoscopy placed in urea solution or jelly. Hp urease releases ammonia which causes a pH change and the yellow indicator turns red	Sensitive (90%), but expense of endoscopy Hp patchily distributed so may result in false-negative test Two biopsies increase sensitivity
Urea breath test	Ingestion of C13 or C14 (radioactive) labelled urea. Hp urease results in cleavage of labelled CO_2 which is then detectable	The most accurate test for diagnosis (98%) (effectively is a test of the whole stomach) and check for successful eradication
Histology	Requires gastric antral biopsy	Seen on haematoxylin and eosin stain but Hp patchy (see CLO test)

Hp, *Helicobacter pylori*.

Drug therapy in gastroenterology

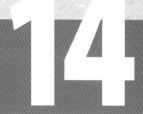

AZATHIOPRINE

14.1 What is the role of azathioprine in gastroenterology?

Azathioprine is a purine analogue which is used to maintain remission or as a steroid-sparing agent in inflammatory bowel disease (ulcerative colitis and Crohn's disease). It is also often used in maintenance of remission of autoimmune hepatitis.

In inflammatory bowel disease the optimal dose is 2–2.5 mg/kg. It is often started at lower doses and titrated upwards.

6-mercaptopurine (6-MP) is the metabolite of azathioprine. It is interchangeable with azathioprine but is used at a lower dose (1.0–1.5 mg/kg). Patients who feel nauseated with azathioprine will often tolerate 6-MP. Historically, azathioprine has been used preferentially in the UK, and 6-MP in the USA.

In Crohn's disease it is used for:

- induction of remission (ARR = 20%, NNT = 5, OR = 2.43 (1.62–3.64)) (Cochrane)
- maintenance of remission (ARR = 15%, NNT = 7, OR = 2.16 (1.35–3.47)) (Cochrane)

In ulcerative colitis (UC) it is used for:

- maintenance of remission – but only weak evidence exists to support its role in the management of UC. In one study patients in remission on azathioprine were randomised to continue with azathioprine or placebo. Significantly more relapsed in the placebo group over the following 12 months.

14.2 What are the main side-effects of azathioprine?

The main side-effects of azathioprine are:

- bone marrow suppression (5%) – almost always reversible on cessation of the drug
- pancreatitis (2–3%) – usually mild and self-limiting on withdrawal of the drug
- a flu-like, hypersensitive reaction, often mild and self-limiting; patients who persevere with the medication may find that this side-effect resolves.

14.3 How should the use of azathioprine be monitored?

Patients started on the drug should have full blood count (FBC) and liver function tests (LFTs) weekly for the first 4 weeks, monthly for 2 months, and then 1–3 monthly thereafter.

They should be advised to stop the drug (or attend for an immediate blood test) if:

■ they experience severe abdominal pain (attend for an amylase to exclude pancreatitis)
■ develop easy bruising or bleeding (attend for a FBC to consider the possibility of thrombocytopenia)
■ develop a severe sore throat or signs of severe sepsis (attend for a FBC to consider the possibility of leucopenia/neutropenia).

Azathioprine is metabolised to 6-mercaptopurine (6-MP), which is further metabolised to the active metabolites, the thioguanine nucleotides (TGNs). TGNs are purine antagonists, and inhibit DNA, RNA and protein synthesis.

Thiopurine methyltransferase (TPMT) is a catabolic enzyme that competes for 6-MP and its nucleotides, converting them into the methylmercaptopurine nucleotides (and therefore diverts 6-MP catabolism away from TGN metabolites). TPMT activity thus has an important effect on the levels of the active metabolite of azathioprine and 6-MP (i.e. TGN); high activity results in low TGN levels and a poorer response to treatment, whereas low or absent TPMT activity leads to high TGN levels and profound myelosuppression.

TPMT activity in the general population is trimodally distributed. The majority of the population (89%) have normal or high levels, 11% have intermediate activity and 0.3% have low activity and are at particular risk of myelosuppression (Lennard 2002). TPMT activity is not yet routinely measured in clinical practice, but there is currently active research in this area.

COLESTYRAMINE

14.4 What is the role of colestyramine in gastroenterology?

Colestyramine is a bile acid binding resin. It is of use in patients with bile salt malabsorption. Secreted bile is normally resorbed in the terminal ileum in a recycling mechanism – the enterohepatic circulation. If this fails to occur, excess bile acids enter the colon, where they are irritant and cause diarrhoea (bile salt diarrhoea). This may occur if the ileum is diseased (e.g. Crohn's disease) or if it has been resected. It may also occur following cholecystectomy, or may be idiopathic. Colestyramine 4 g once to three times per day (or colestipol) binds bile and prevents its irritant effect on the colon.

Colestyramine is also used to relieve the pruritus associated with primary biliary cirrhosis (rifampicin can also be used in this respect).

14.5 What are the side-effects of colestyramine?

It may produce gastrointestinal side-effects. In addition, the bile acid binding resins may interfere with fat-soluble vitamin absorption (vitamins A, D, E and K) and supplementation may be necessary in prolonged use. Since these resins may also bind other drugs and interfere with absorption, other medications should be taken either 1 hour before the resin or 4–6 hours afterwards.

14.6 How should the use of colestyramine be monitored?

No routine blood tests are required.

INTERFERON

14.7 What is the role of interferon in gastroenterology?

Interferon is used to clear chronic hepatitis B and C virus infection.

Interferon alpha may clear hepatitis B virus in less than 40% of patients. Interferon alpha plus ribavirin clears hepatitis C virus in approximately 40% of patients (compared to less than 20% if interferon is used alone). More recently, pegylated (a slow release formulation) alpha interferon (in association with ribavirin) has been introduced for chronic hepatitis C treatment and produces better results (overall approximately 55% of patients have a sustained virological response). Response rate depends on the hepatitis C genotype. Genotypes 2 and 3 have up to 80% sustained virological response (after 6 months of interferon treatment), whereas genotype 1 response is around 50% (after 12 months of interferon treatment).

14.8 What are the side-effects of interferon/ribavirin therapy?

Lethargy and influenza-like symptoms are common side-effects of interferon, and may be problematic, especially in younger patients with children (and the attendant responsibilities). Other problems include depression, myelosuppression and hepatic and renal toxicity. Occasionally, autoimmune disease may be triggered (e.g. thyroid problems).

The main side-effect of ribavirin is haemolytic anaemia, and may necessitate a dose reduction in about one-fifth of patients treated. Ribavirin is teratogenic and pregnancy should be avoided while on treatment and for 6 months afterwards for women on treatment and for partners of men on treatment.

14.9 How should interferon therapy be monitored?

Patients should have full blood count, biochemistry, glucose and urate monitored monthly; thyroid function should also be checked periodically (e.g. 3 monthly).

METHOTREXATE

14.10 What is the role of methotrexate in gastroenterology?

This is a useful drug in the treatment of steroid-refractory or steroid-dependent Crohn's disease, usually used if azathioprine fails or the patient is intolerant to azathioprine.

It is given as a once-weekly 25 mg intramuscular injection for 16 weeks. Oral administration is not as reliable, especially if the patient has small bowel disease, because of problems of variable absorption. A single double-blind randomised controlled trial showed 39% of patients were able to wean off prednisolone completely and remain in clinical remission compared to 19% given placebo (Feagan et al 1995). A follow-up study on those who had achieved remission showed that 15 mg methotrexate given intramuscularly once weekly for a further 40 weeks was able to successfully maintain remission in 65% versus 39% on placebo (Feagan et al 2000).

14.11 What are the main side-effects of methotrexate?

 It may cause stomatitis, diarrhoea, hair loss and leucopenia. Transaminitis may occur. Interstitial pneumonitis is a rare but potentially life-threatening side-effect.

14.12 How should the use of methotrexate be monitored?

 Patients started on the drug should:

- ■ have a FBC and LFTs weekly for the first 4 weeks, then monthly thereafter
- ■ be warned about the onset of cough or shortness of breath
- ■ be advised about the teratogenic effects of methotrexate; females of child-bearing age must use a highly effective contraceptive.

PROPRANOLOL

14.13 What is the role of propranolol in gastroenterology?

There is clear evidence for the use of propranolol in both primary and secondary prophylaxis of oesophageal variceal bleeds (Jalan & Hayes 2000). Propranolol has been shown to reduce the risk of a first variceal bleed, and there is a trend towards a decrease in mortality (Poynard et al 1991, D'Amico et al 1999).

The aim of therapy is to reduce the portal pressure gradient (and hence the pressure within the varices themselves) to <12 mmHg. The portal pressure (as measured via a balloon catheter wedged into the hepatic vein) is rarely used in clinical practice, and a currently used surrogate marker is a reduction in the resting pulse of 25%. Propranolol is usually started at a dose of 40 mg bd and increased to 80 mg bd if necessary.

If propranolol is contraindicated or not tolerated, variceal band ligation is recommended. Isosorbide mononitrate is an alternative at a dosage of 20 mg bd, if neither propranolol nor band ligation is possible.

Similar results have been shown with propranolol in the prevention of recurrent variceal bleeding and a reduction in mortality (secondary prophylaxis), following endoscopic obliteration of varices.

14.14 What are the side-effects of propranolol?

These comprise the usual side-effects of non-selective beta-blockers.

14.15 How should propranolol therapy be monitored?

Propranolol itself needs no monitoring.

URSODEOXYCHOLIC ACID

14.16 What is the role of ursodeoxycholic acid in gastroenterology?

Ursodeoxycholic acid is a hydrophilic bile acid that is present in very small quantities in normal bile. Treatment with ursodeoxycholic acid increases its level within serum and bile from <5% up to 30–60% of total bile acids. The mechanism underlying its potentially beneficial effect in the treatment of primary biliary cirrhosis (PBC) is not completely known.

It is used commonly in the treatment of PBC and results in an improvement in liver biochemistry in patients with this disorder. A meta-analysis has thrown doubt on its benefit in the treatment of PBC (Goulis et al 1999); however, different doses of ursodeoxycholic acid were used in different patient populations. A pooled analysis of three double-blind randomised trials in which an equivalent dose of ursodeoxycholic acid was used (13–15 mg/kg) showed a significant increase in the time free from liver transplantation over a 4-year treatment period in the ursodeoxycholic acid treated patients compared to placebo (Poupon et al 1997). Some of the placebo group in two of the trials were switched to ursodeoxycholic acid, but analysis was based on intention-to-treat, i.e. analysed as if they were still on placebo. This 'partially treated group' within the placebo group would, if anything, have likely lessened any potential differences between treatment and placebo groups, making it more likely that ursodeoxycholic acid is indeed beneficial.

It is also often used in the treatment of primary sclerosing cholangitis (a much rarer condition). It will often improve liver biochemistry, but it is unclear whether it exerts any beneficial effect on the natural history of the disease.

Its other potential use is in the dissolution of gallstones. Its mechanism of action is to desaturate bile and cholesterol, and it may do this by reducing the intestinal absorption of cholesterol.

Bile acid dissolution therapy should be reserved for those with uncomplicated (cholesterol) gallstones (i.e. not those with acute cholecystitis, cholangitis, pancreatitis or common bile duct obstruction). Symptoms, in those suitable for treatment, should be mild and infrequent. Approximately 80% of gallstones are cholesterol gallstones.

An oral cholecystogram was formerly employed to reveal whether a gallbladder was functioning (i.e. able to concentrate bile) and also to determine whether the cystic duct was patent – both prerequisites to successful gallstone dissolution therapy. However, 'functional ultrasound scans' – which show emptying of the gallbladder in response to a meal, patency of the cystic duct and complications of gallbladder disease – are increasingly being used.

Bile acid dissolution therapy works best in radiolucent stones (therefore more likely to be cholesterol stones) less than 5 mm in diameter. Ursodeoxycholic acid in a dose of 10–15 mg/kg per day dissolves 20–70% of stones. A recent meta-analysis of dissolution trials showed an overall dissolution success of 37% (<5 mm stones = >70%; <10 mm stones = 49%; >10 mm stones = 29%) (May et al 1993). Duration of therapy depends on the size of the stone and varies between 6 and 18 months. It may be required long term, since stones may reform in approximately 25% of patients within 1 year of cessation of treatment.

14.17 What are the side-effects of ursodeoxycholic acid?

 It is extremely safe and virtually devoid of side-effects. A few people may suffer from diarrhoea or vomiting, but it causes no problem in the vast majority.

14.18 How should the use of ursodeoxycholic acid be monitored?

The *British National Formulary* suggests caution in its use in liver disease; clinically, however, it is usually prescribed in the treatment of PBC.

There is no particular requirement for periodic blood testing (LFTs will of course be performed routinely in the outpatient management of those with PBC).

5-AMINOSALICYLATES

14.19 What is the role of 5-aminosalicylates in gastroenterology?

The 5-aminosalicylates sulfasalazine and mesalazine are useful in the treatment and maintenance of remission of ulcerative colitis. The evidence of usefulness is much weaker for Crohn's disease.

■ *Sulfasalazine* – the first agent and as effective as the newer preparations, but has a greater incidence of side-effects. It consists of a carrier molecule, sulfapyridine (which is the cause of the side-effects), linked by an azo bond to the active moiety, 5-aminosalicylic acid (5-ASA). Colonic bacteria cleave the bond and release active 5-ASA in the colon. It is a second-line agent in the treatment of rheumatoid arthritis and may be useful in those patients with inflammatory bowel disease who have an associated arthropathy.

The newer preparations consist of either 5-ASA alone with targeted delivery to the small and or large bowel, or employ an alternative carrier molecule to sulfapyridine.

■ *Asacol, Salofalk* – 5-ASA coated in a pH-sensitive resin designed to release in the ileocaecal region.
■ *Pentasa* – 5-ASA in a semi-permeable membrane releases 5-ASA throughout the small and large bowel. It is therefore the 5-ASA of choice if used in small bowel Crohn's disease.
■ *Olsalazine, balsalazide* – 5-ASA linked to 5-ASA (olsalazine) or a peptide (balsalazide).

All of these drugs are generic 'mesalazine' and represent one of the rare situations in medicine when prescribing by trade name may be more appropriate given that their release mechanisms and therefore sites of action are different.

14.20 What are the side-effects of 5-aminosalicylates?

These drugs are generally very well tolerated and side-effects are relatively rare, especially with the newer salicylates.

Sulfasalazine may cause the usual side-effects associated with sulphonamide antibiotics due to its sulfapyridine molecule. These include bone marrow suppression, liver abnormalities, nausea and vomiting, rash and erythema nodosum. These problems are not generally seen with the other aminosalicylates but they may still cause skin rash, nausea and diarrhoea.

Potentially the most serious side-effect of the newer 5-ASA drugs is renal damage due to an interstitial nephritis. This is, in fact, very rare and the need for monitoring is much debated.

14.21 How should the use of 5-aminosalicylates be monitored?

Sulfasalazine patients should have FBC and LFTs monitored 3–6 monthly. Monitoring of the newer 5-ASAs is not well established. The authors recommend 6–12 monthly monitoring of serum urea and electrolytes and dip-sticking of urine. This can often be achieved during routine follow-up in an inflammatory bowel disease clinic.

HISTAMINE-2 RECEPTOR ANTAGONISTS

14.22 What is the role of histamine-2 receptor antagonists in gastroenterology?

The histamine-2 receptor antagonists (H2RAs) cimetidine, ranitidine, famotidine and nizatidine are useful acid suppressants. They have, by and large, been superseded by the proton pump inhibitors, especially in the treatment of gastro-oesophageal reflux disease. Although PPIs inhibit the final common pathway in gastric acid production (i.e. irreversibly bind to the proton pump), they are not completely efficacious. In patients with particularly troublesome nocturnal reflux symptoms, despite PPI therapy, the addition of a small dose of a H2RA (e.g. ranitidine 150 mg) at bedtime can be highly effective (by inhibiting a specific acid-promoting pathway).

14.23 What are the side-effects of histamine-2 receptor antagonists?

H2RAs are well tolerated but may cause gastrointestinal disturbances, including diarrhoea. Headaches, dizziness, rash and altered liver function tests are also reported.

It is worth noting that cimetidine inhibits the cytochrome p450 system, and therefore may potentiate the action of drugs such as warfarin, anticonvulsants and theophylline. Cimetidine also has anti-androgen properties, and may cause gynaecomastia.

14.24 How should the use of histamine-2 receptor antagonists be monitored?

There is no requirement for specific blood test monitoring, unless the patient develops particular symptoms which dictate further investigation.

PROKINETIC DRUGS

14.25 What is the role of prokinetic drugs in gastroenterology?

Metoclopramide and domperidone, both dopamine antagonists, are employed chiefly as anti-emetics. They accelerate gastric emptying and small bowel transit, and increase lower oesophageal sphincter tone.

Excepting their roles as anti-emetics, the evidence for the efficacy of metoclopramide (or domperidone) as an effective agent in gastro-oesophageal reflux disease, either alone or in combination with a H2RA, is minimal.

14.26 What are the side-effects of the prokinetic drugs?

 Metoclopramide and domperidone are usually very well tolerated. Both may cause acute dystonic reactions, but this is less likely with domperidone which does not cross the blood–brain barrier so easily.

Cisapride (a 5HT3 antagonist and partial 5HT4 agonist) is equivalent to H2RAs in symptom control and healing of minor grades of oesophagitis, but has been withdrawn from general use because of its cardiotoxic side-effects (QT interval prolongation, ventricular arrhythmias and death).

14.27 How should the use of prokinetic drugs be monitored?

No routine blood tests are required.

PROTON PUMP INHIBITORS

14.28 What is the role of proton pump inhibitors in gastroenterology?

The proton pump inhibitors (PPIs) omeprazole, lansoprazole, rabeprazole, pantoprazole and esomeprazole are powerful acid suppressants which work on the hydrogen–potassium–ATPase pump, the final common pathway in acid production by the parietal cell. All are highly effective in ulcer healing and treatment of erosive oesophagitis.

It is difficult to make meaningful comparisons between the five PPIs as treatment and healing dose strengths differ amongst the different PPIs. Rabeprazole and pantoprazole have fewer drug interactions (e.g. no effect on warfarin or phenytoin). Esomeprazole (the purified S isomer of omeprazole) 40 mg daily is more effective at healing more severe grades of oesophagitis than lansoprazole 30 mg daily.

Current NICE guidance (2000) suggests that the cheapest, lowest effective dose of PPI should be used where possible.

14.29 What are the side-effects of proton pump inhibitors?

 PPIs are very safe drugs with few documented side-effects. There may be an increase in the incidence of enteric infections in patients who take these medications long term. Initial early fears linking PPI use to the development of gastric carcinoma have so far proved unfounded. These concerns arose largely because of the link between other prolonged states of profound hypochlorhydria (pernicious anaemia, duodenal ulcer surgery) and gastric cancer. Nevertheless, many gastroenterologists would recommend alternative management approaches in young patients (under 50) needing long-term PPI therapy if such alternatives are available – for example, laparoscopic fundoplication for oesophageal reflux disease.

14.30 How should the use of proton pump inhibitors be monitored?

These drugs do not need any particular monitoring.

OTHER DRUGS

14.31 What is the role of amitriptyline in gastroenterology?

Amitriptyline is a tricyclic antidepressant used in low dose for irritable bowel syndrome patients who have predominant pain which is not ameliorated by reassurance and antispasmodics. The usual dosage is 10–25 mg, although this may be increased into the conventional antidepressant dosage range as coexistent mood disorders are not uncommon.

14.32 What is the role of budesonide in gastroenterology?

This is an alternative steroid to prednisolone (*see* Q 14.36). It is more potent and undergoes almost complete first pass metabolism through the liver, thereby reducing the systemic side-effects of steroids. Budesonide 9 mg per day was comparable to prednisolone 40 mg per day in the treatment of active Crohn's disease (Rutgeerts et al 1994). It has also been shown to be as efficacious as prednisolone in the treatment of ulcerative colitis (Lofberg et al 1996). It is much more expensive than prednisolone.

14.33 What is the role of ciclosporin in gastroenterology?

It is used as an infusion for severe ulcerative colitis unresponsive to 5–7 days of intravenous hydrocortisone. Formerly the only option for such patients was a colectomy. A small double-blind, randomised, controlled trial of just 20 patients failing to respond to 7–10 days of intravenous hydrocortisone showed that over 80% of patients given ciclosporin achieved remission versus 0% in the placebo group (Lichtiger et al 1994). Since then, other reports show a success rate of 60–65%, but with many patients who respond requiring a colectomy within the next 12 months. It is nevertheless useful, especially in patients with a first attack who have yet to try or be maintained on azathioprine.

14.34 What is the role of infliximab in gastroenterology?

Infliximab (anti-tumour necrosis factor antibody) is the newest addition to drug therapy for Crohn's disease. It is given as an infusion as a day case in the hospital setting. It has been shown to improve disease activity in approximately 65% of patients with moderate to severe Crohn's, and to put one-third into remission (Targan et al 1997). It has also been shown to have a beneficial effect on enterocutaneous (mostly perianal in the trial) fistula, with over half showing complete healing (Present et al 1999).

Transfusion reactions and progressive decrease in effectiveness can both be signs of antibody formation against the drug. These may be limited by concomitant administration of immunosuppressants, usually methotrexate or azathioprine.

Initially, infliximab was used in gastroenterology as a remission-inducing treatment, given as a course of three doses. There is an increasing trend to use it as maintenance therapy, giving the drug every 8–12 weeks over many months. This usage follows the example of its use in rheumatology, where the drug is extensively prescribed for patients with inflammatory arthritides.

Oral preparations are in development but the biggest challenge facing this drug, whether oral or intravenous, is cost: each infusion costs up to £1000.

14.35 What is the role of metronidazole in gastroenterology?

Metronidazole is useful in perianal Crohn's disease. It is usually only used for a period of 6 weeks or so because of the increasing incidence of peripheral neuropathy thereafter.

It is also used as a first line agent for the treatment of *Clostridium difficile* infection (pseudomembranous colitis) which may complicate antibiotic treatments. It is given for 7–10 days. If this is unsuccessful or the infection recurs shortly afterwards, oral vancomycin 125 mg qds is a frequently used alternative. Either is effective, but metronidazole is cheaper.

14.36 What is the role of prednisolone in gastroenterology?

This is the main treatment of acute flare-ups of ulcerative colitis or Crohn's disease. It is also used in the management of autoimmune hepatitis. Generally speaking, an initial dose of 30–40 mg per day is tapered by 5 mg per day at 1–2 weekly intervals.

14.37 What is the role of terlipressin in gastroenterology?

Terlipressin (Glypressin) is a synthetic analogue of vasopressin, but has less effect on peripheral resistance and cardiac status. It is used as a vasoconstrictor (of the splanchnic blood flow) in the setting of an acute variceal bleed, and is given as an intravenous injection. It may also have a role in the reversal/prevention of hepatorenal syndrome.

OTHER THERAPIES

14.38 What is 'triple therapy'?

Triple therapy refers to the combination of high dose PPI (e.g. omeprazole 40 mg bd, lansoprazole 30 mg bd, etc.) with two of three antibiotics (clarithromycin 500 mg bd, amoxicillin 1 g bd or metronidazole 400 mg bd). The combination is highly effective at eradicating *Helicobacter pylori* in around 90% of patients (*see Ch. 2*)

14.39 What is 'quadruple therapy'?

If triple therapy fails, quadruple therapy may be tried. This is a more complex regimen with four drugs with different dosing schedules administered over a period of 2 weeks in total. It consists of omeprazole 40 mg bd, tripotassium dicitratobismuthate (De-Nol) 1 tab qds, metronidazole 400 mg tds and tetracycline 500 mg qds.

Appendix 2 lists many of the commonly used drugs in gastroenterological practice. It is not an exhaustive guide of either the drugs themselves or their many potential side-effects, but hopefully summarises the main indications and contains useful information on usual dosages and treatment regimens, and notes on clinical practice/evidence.

FERTILITY AND PREGNANCY

14.40 How does inflammatory bowel disease influence fertility and pregnancy, and what are the risks of the medications commonly taken?

A frequent and difficult question arises in the use of medications during pregnancy. Ideally, although no drug should be taken during pregnancy, it is important to weigh up the risks of the particular medication (for the treatment of active disease, or maintenance of remission) against the risks of not treating active disease and the likely increased risks of relapse if the maintenance treatment is discontinued. There needs to be an informed discussion with the patient and a plan agreed on an individual basis.

Many patients suffering from inflammatory bowel disease are of child-bearing age, and a substantial proportion are maintained on 5-ASAs or immunosuppressive therapy (azathioprine or 6-mercaptopurine). The dilemma is whether to advise stopping these drugs preconceptually or during pregnancy with the attendant risk of relapse, which also may adversely affect birth outcome.

Women who develop inflammatory bowel disease before their first pregnancy have fewer children compared to population controls. Women with inflammatory bowel disease also have a significant risk of having a preterm delivery (<37 weeks) and a low birth weight baby (<2500g) (Alstead et al 2003).

Many patients, especially those with ulcerative colitis, will be maintained on 5-ASAs. A cohort study from Denmark examined the risk of malformations (in mothers prescribed 5-ASAs in the 30 days prior to conception to the end of the first trimester – 'early pregnancy') and stillbirths, preterm births, and low birth weights (in mothers prescribed 5-ASAs during the first to third trimesters – 'entire pregnancy') compared to controls. The principal results are summarised in *Table 14.1*.

The odds ratio of these events occurring in mothers prescribed 5-ASAs (overall, 5-ASA alone, or 5-ASA plus steroid) compared to controls are summarised in *Table 14.2*.

Furthermore, on stratifying for disease (either Crohn's or ulcerative colitis), it was found that the risk for preterm birth and stillbirth was only present in the mothers with ulcerative colitis who had been prescribed 5-ASAs compared to controls (*Table 14.3*).

It could, however, be that it is the disease process itself, rather than the medication, that is responsible for the increase in adverse birth outcomes. A comparison was therefore made between mothers with inflammatory bowel disease (IBD) prescribed 5-ASAs during pregnancy and IBD controls (not exposed to 5-ASAs in pregnancy) (*Table 14.4*).

TABLE 14.1 Birth outcome in patients treated with 5-aminosalicylic acid (5-ASA) in pregnancy compared to controls

	'Early' pregnancy (n=60) Events (%)	'Entire' pregnancy (n=88) Events (%)	Controls (n=19 418) Events (%)
Stillbirths	2 (3.3)	3 (3.4)	109 (0.6)
Malformations	4 (6.7)	5 (5.7)	711 (3.7)
Preterm birth	6 (10.0)	8 (9.1)	1062 (5.5)

Data from Norgard et al (2003), with permission.

TABLE 14.2 Birth outcome in patients treated with 5-aminosalicylic acid (5-ASA) in pregnancy, stratified for concomitant use of steroids

	5-ASA alone (n=61)	5-ASA ± steroid (overall) (n=88)	5-ASA + steroid (n=27)
Stillbirths	2.8 (0.3–23.8)	6.4 (1.7–24.9)	20.4 (3.4–122.9)
Malformations	1.3 (0.3–5.3)	1.9 (0.7–5.4)	3.9 (0.9–17.2)
Preterm birth	2.4 (1.1–5.3)	1.9 (0.9–3.9)	0.8 (0.1–5.7)

Numerical values are odds ratio, with 95% confidence intervals in parentheses.
Data from Norgard et al (2003), with permission.

TABLE 14.3 Birth outcome in patients treated with 5-aminosalicylic acid (5-ASA) in pregnancy, stratified by type of underlying disease

	Crohn's disease (*n*=23)	Ulcerative colitis (*n*=65)
Stillbirths	n/a (no stillbirths)	8.4 (2.0–34.3)
Malformations	1.5 (0.2–11.4)	2.1 (0.7–6.9)
Preterm birth	0.8 (0.1–5.6)	2.4 (1.1–5.3)

Numerical values are odds ratio, with 95% confidence intervals in parentheses.
Data from Norgard et al (2003), with permission.

TABLE 14.4 Birth outcome in patients treated with 5-aminosalicylic acid (5-ASA) in pregnancy, compared with a control IBD group not exposed to 5-ASA in pregnancy

	IBD exposed events/total (%)	IBD control events/total (%)	Odds ratio (95% CI)
Stillbirths	3/88 (3.4)	2/243 (0.8)	7.1 (0.2–205.1)
Malformations	4/60 (6.7)	10/243 (4.1)	1.5 (0.4–5.1)
Preterm birth	8/88 (9.1)	14/243 (5.8)	2.0 (0.8–5.0)

Data from Norgard et al (2003), with permission.

What can we learn from this study? The first point to make is that the numbers of women exposed to 5-ASAs during pregnancy is relatively low, and because the events are uncommon the confidence intervals are very wide and almost all cross 1 (making the validity of a truly raised odds ratio questionable). That said, there does appear to be an increased risk of stillbirth, malformations and preterm birth in patients exposed to 5-ASAs who suffer from ulcerative colitis. The finding of an increased risk of these adverse birth outcomes when the exposed mothers are compared with IBD controls suggests an association with 5-ASA use, but it may equally reflect disease activity in this group and this factor might be responsible for the adverse outcomes. A similar explanation may be made for the increased risk of stillbirths seen in those treated with 5-ASA and steroids (i.e. it could implicate steroids, but equally may reflect the adverse effect of disease activity) (Norgard et al 2003).

Since the evidence for 5-ASA maintenance in Crohn's disease is weak, one might suggest that the drug is stopped in those women planning to start a family. The issue with women suffering from ulcerative colitis is more complicated, and will depend on how difficult their disease is to manage, together with a careful discussion of the facts with the patient.

A recent retrospective study showed no adverse effect of 6-mercaptopurine (6-MP), the metabolite of azathioprine, on pregnancy. The results of 325 pregnancies in 155 patients (79 females, 76 males) were studied. The successful outcome of pregnancy (i.e. without spontaneous abortion, elective abortion secondary to a birth defect, ectopic pregnancy, anembryonic pregnancy, embryonic demise, major congenital abnormality, neoplasm, or severe or frequent infections) was no different in patients exposed to 6-MP (6-MP stopped before conception: 84 conceptions; after conception: 61 pregnancies; or continued throughout pregnancy: 15 pregnancies) compared to control IBD patients (165 pregnancies) who had never been exposed to 6-MP. The relative rate of successful pregnancy outcome was 0.85 (95% CI, 0.47–1.55). It is noteworthy that major congenital abnormalities occurred in just 2.4% of live births in patients exposed to 6-MP compared to 4% of the IBD controls (Francella et al 2003). Major congenital abnormalities in infants in the general population occur in approximately 2% of individuals.

The recent British Society of Gastroenterology guidelines on inflammatory bowel disease advise that conception should take place during remission and that maintenance medication should be continued. Acute severe colitis should be managed as for non-pregnant patients, since the best interests of the foetus are served by optimal management of the mother's disease. Steroids can be used for active disease, and in general azathioprine should be continued during pregnancy since the risks to the foetus from disease activity are likely to be greater than that from azathioprine (Carter et al 2004).

Chemotherapy in gastrointestinal tract cancers

15

15.1 How is colorectal carcinoma staged?

Colorectal cancer (CRC) is the fourth commonest malignancy in the world, accounting for over 1 million new cases and over 500 000 deaths per year. In the UK, it is the third most common cancer, affecting over 30 000 people each year, and is the second most common cause of cancer-related death. The average 5-year survival is approximately 40%.

The most important prognostic factor is the pathological stage at presentation, with the depth of invasion of the tumour into the bowel wall and the degree of involvement of regional lymph nodes the principal determinants. The original Dukes staging system has now been superseded by the TNM (tumour–node–metastasis) classification (*Table 15.1*).

15.2 I have a patient who has just been diagnosed with colorectal cancer and liver metastases. What is their prognosis?

The presence of liver metastases complicating colorectal carcinoma does not necessarily mean that the patient is incurable. In selected cases, where there are solitary or only a few metastases, or the metastatic deposits are restricted in lobar distribution, resection of the primary lesion and metastatic deposit can result in a 5-year survival of approximately 30%. Unfortunately, the presence of liver metastases often renders the patient incurable.

Without treatment, the median survival is approximately 6 months. Treatment with fluorouracil (and leucovorin, which stabilises the binding of fluorouracil to thymidylate synthase) approximately doubles median survival to around 11 months.

Fluorouracil (5-FU) is usually administered intravenously because of erratic bioavailability when taken orally (thought to be due to variable individual intestinal mucosal concentrations of its catabolic enzyme, dihydropyrimidine dehydrogenase). Recently, an oral prodrug, capecitabine (Xeloda), which is absorbed intact and then converted to fluorouracil, has been approved by the US Food and Drug Administration (FDA). In randomised trials it has shown equivalence to monthly intravenous therapy with fluorouracil and leucovorin (median survival 12–13 months).

The combination of other cytotoxics to fluorouracil therapy has been shown to further increase median survival. The addition of oxaliplatin and irinotecan (either in combination, or sequentially) to intravenous fluorouracil and leucovorin regimens has been shown to extend median survival times to 19–21 months.

TABLE 15.1 Tumour-node-metastasis classification

Stage	TNM classification	5-year survival (%)
I	T1–2, N0, M0	>90
IIA	T3, N0, M0	60–85
IIB	T4, N0, M0	
IIIA	T1–2, N1, M0	
IIIB	T3–4, N1, M0	25–65
IIIC	T(any), N2, M0	
IV	T(any), N(any), M1	5–7

T1 = tumour invades submucosa
T2 = tumour invades muscle layers
T3 = tumour through muscle layers and into subserosa
T4 = tumour invades into organ/structure or perforates visceral peritoneum
N0 = no regional lymph node involvement
N1 = metastases present in 1–3 regional lymph nodes
N2 = metastases in ≥4 regional lymph nodes
M0 = no distant metastases
M1 = distant metastases.

15.3 What does the future hold for chemotherapy in metastatic colorectal disease?

Recently two further 'targeted' drugs have been approved by the FDA for the management of advanced colorectal cancer:

■ Cetuximab (Erbitux) is a monoclonal antibody directed against the epidermal growth factor receptor (important in pathways regulating cell growth, proliferation, and apoptosis).

■ Bevacizumab (Avastin) is an antibody directed against vascular endothelial growth factor, which is important in angiogenesis. The addition of bevacizumab to irinotecan and fluorouracil/leucovorin regimens improved median survival time to 20.3 months, compared to 15.6 months (irinotecan and fluorouracil/leucovorin plus placebo).

Efforts are now being made to tailor chemotherapeutic regimens to individual patients. This is likely to be easier when the various genetic polymorphisms affecting the metabolism of individual chemotherapeutic agents have been elucidated, and similarly the biological pathways of the 'targeted' drugs.

15.4 Do any of the chemotherapeutic agents improve survival when used in conjunction with potentially curative resection (adjuvant/neoadjuvant chemotherapy)?

Intravenous fluorouracil ± leucovorin adjuvant therapy improves the prognosis of stage III disease (i.e. lymph node positive disease). Pooled analyses have shown that 5-year survival is improved from 51 to 64%. Oral and intravenous fluoropyrimidines seem equally efficacious. By contrast, postoperative fluoropyrimidine treatment in stage II disease (T3–4 but lymph node negative) appears to offer no significant survival advantage (Meyerhardt & Mayer 2005).

15.5 What side-effects can I expect from chemotherapy?

Most regimens involve the fluoropyrimidines, and the side-effects depend on how they are given. The side-effects, as with many chemotherapeutic agents, include diarrhoea, nausea, vomiting and suppression of the immune system.

The commonest side-effects when fluorouracil is given as a 'loading' schedule (i.e. given intravenously on a daily basis for five consecutive days at monthly intervals) are a sore mouth (stomatitis) and suppression of the immune system (neutropenia). If given intravenously once a week, diarrhoea is a more common side-effect.

Fluorouracil is sometimes given by continuous intravenous infusion; this results in less chance of immune suppression and a sore mouth, but the palms of the hands and soles of the feet may become red and sore ('hand–foot syndrome'). The most common side-effect with oral fluorouracil is the hand–foot syndrome.

15.6 What is the role of chemo/radiotherapy in the palliation of incurable oesophageal adenocarcinoma?

Unfortunately, it is only in about 20% of patients with oesophageal adenocarcinomas that surgery is able to provide prolonged survival. If very early tumours are detected (T1, confined to the mucosa/submucosa), 5-year survival is 50–80% following surgical resection. Sadly, the majority of oesophageal carcinomas present at a much later stage, when treatment is palliative. The most immediate concern is usually to improve dysphagia, and this may be achieved by placement of expandable metal stents, or laser therapy.

Chemoradiation appears to confer survival advantage over radiotherapy alone, improving median survival from 8.9 to 12.5 months (Herskovic et al 1992).

15.7 What is the role of chemo/radiotherapy in the palliation of incurable gastric and gastro-oesophageal junction adenocarcinoma?

Chemotherapy improves quality of life and survival in gastric and gastro-oesophageal junction adenocarcinomas. Epirubicin, cisplatin and continuous 5-FU infusion (ECF) is a preferred option, resulting in a survival time of 8.9 months compared to 5.7 months with FAMTX (5-FU, adriamycin, methotrexate), and a significantly better 2-year survival rate (13.5% versus 5.4%).

15.8 Does chemo/radiotherapy improve survival when used in conjunction with potentially curative oesophageal resection (adjuvant/neoadjuvant chemotherapy)?

Currently, postoperative chemotherapy after oesophageal resection does not significantly improve overall 5-year survival.

Neoadjuvant chemotherapy with preoperative cisplatin and 5-FU showed a significant survival improvement over surgery alone, with a median survival of 530 versus 408 days (UK Medical Research Council OEO2 Trial – unpublished data).

Preoperative radiotherapy has not been shown to confer benefit.

A meta-analysis of five trials has shown a small but significant 3-year survival benefit from combined preoperative chemo- and radiotherapy (31%) versus surgery alone (22%) (Allum et al 2002).

15.9 Does chemo/radiotherapy improve survival when used in conjunction with potentially curative gastro-oesophageal/gastric resection (adjuvant/neoadjuvant chemotherapy)?

There is currently insufficient evidence to recommend pre- or postoperative chemotherapy or chemo/radiotherapy after gastric or gastro-oesophageal carcinoma resection.

15.10 Is chemo/radiotherapy as good as surgery for squamous cell oesophageal carcinoma?

Squamous cell oesophageal carcinomas usually arise in the mid/proximal oesophagus and may represent a greater surgical challenge. Combined chemo/radiotherapy alone can be curative and seems to be equivalent to surgery, with cure rates above 20% (Allum et al 2002).

15.11 What palliation is available for inoperable hepatocellular carcinoma?

The only curative procedure for hepatocellular carcinoma (HCC) is either resection of tumour (one lesion ≤5 cm or up to three lesions each ≤3 cm) or transplantation (if the liver is cirrhotic) with identical criteria (Ryder 2003).

Palliative techniques include percutaneous ethanol injection (PEI) and 5-year survival rates of 35–75% are reported. There is a lack of randomised studies, but against historical controls PEI looks as good as surgery and so seems certainly to be the best option for small inoperable HCCs. Radiofrequency ablation is a newer alternative technique.

There is currently no role for intravenous chemotherapy.

GP and patient information

Beating Bowel Cancer
39 Crown Road
St Margarets
Twickenham TW1 3EJ
Tel: 0208 892 5256
Fax: 0208 892 1008
www.bowelcancer.org

British Colostomy Association
15 Station Road
Reading RG1 1LG
Helpline: 0800 328 4257
Tel: 01189 391 537
Fax: 01189 569 095
www.bcass.org.uk

British Liver Trust
Portman House
44 High Street
Ringwood
Hampshire BH24 1AG
Tel: 01425 463080
Email: info@britishlivertrust.org.uk
www.britishlivertrust.org.uk

Coeliac UK
PO Box 220
High Wycombe
Buckinghamshire HP11 2HY
Helpline: 0870 444 8804 (10.00–16.00 Mon–Fri)
Tel (Admin): 01494 437278
Fax: 01494 474349
www.coeliac.co.uk

Colon Cancer Concern
Tel (Infoline): 08708 50 60 50
www.coloncancer.org.uk

CORE (Digestive Disorders Foundation)
3 St Andrew's Place
London NW1 4LB
Tel: 0207 486 0341
Fax: 0207 224 2012
www.corecharity.org.uk

Expert Panel of Advice on the Diagnosis and Management of Ulcerative Colitis and Crohn's Disease for GPs
R Jones, D Jewel and J Price
c/o Hyde Lodge
Hyde Lane
Churt
Surrey GU10 2LP
Tel: 01428 604444

Gut Motility Disorders Support Network
Tel: 01398 351173

The Hepatitis C Trust
27 Crosby Row
London SE1 3YD
Helpline: 0870 200 1200
Email: info@hepctrust.org
www.hepcuk.info

ia (Ileostomy and Internal Pouch Support Group)
Peverill House
1–5 Mill Road
Ballyclare
Co. Antrim
Northern Ireland BT39 9DR
Tel: 0800 018 4724
http://the-ia.org.uk

Irritable Bowel Syndrome (IBS) Network
Unit 5, 53 Mowbray Street
Sheffield S3 8EN
Helpline: 0114 272 3253 (18.00–20.00 Mon–Fri; 10.00–12.00 Sat)
www.ibsnetwork.org.uk

National Association for Colitis and Crohn's Disease (UK)
4 Beaumont House
Sutton Road
St Albans
Herts AL1 5HH
Tel (Information): 0845 130 2233
Tel (Admin): 01727 830038
Fax: 01727 862550
www.nacc.org.uk

National Hepatitis C Resource Centre
PO Box 31844
London SE11 4DT
Advice Line: 0870 242 2467
Email: info@hepccentre.org.uk
www.hepccentre.org.uk

Oesophageal Patients Association
22 Vulcan House, Vulcan Road
Solihull B91 2JY
Tel: 0121 704 9860 (09.00–17.00, Mon–Fri)
www.opa.org.uk

Pancreatitis Supporters' Network
PO Box 8938
Birmingham B13 9FW
Tel/fax: 0121 449 0667
www.pancreatitis.org.uk

PINNT (Patients on Intravenous and Naso-gastric Nutrition Therapy)
PO Box 3126
Christchurch
Dorset BH23 2XS
Tel/fax: 01202 481 625
www.pinnt.com

Informative websites
- Bandolier: **www.jr2.ox.ac.uk/bandolier**
- Big Matters: **www.bigmatters.co.uk**
- British Medical Journal (clinical evidence website):
  www.clinicalevidence.com
- British Medical Journal (learning website): **www.bmjlearning.com**
- British Medical Journal: **www.bmj.com**

- British National Formulary: www.bnf.org
- British Nutrition Foundation: www.nutrition.org.uk
- British Society of Gastroenterology: www.bsg.org.uk
- CancerBACUP: www.cancerbacup.org.uk
- Department of Health: www.dh.gov.uk
- Education website for doctors: www.doctors.net.uk
- Health Protection Agency: www.hpa.org.uk
- National Electronic Library for Health (clinical evidence website): www.nelh.nhs.uk/clinical_evidence.asp
- National Health Service (diet and nutrition sites): www.5ADAY.nhs.uk; www.eatwell.gov.uk
- National Health Service Hepatitis C information line: www.hepc.nhs.uk
- National Health Service Information Authority: www.nhsia.nhs.uk
- National Institute for Health and Clinical Excellence (NICE): www.nice.org.uk
- National Obesity Forum: www.nationalobesityforum.org.uk
- National Prescribing Centre: www.npc.co.uk
- Obesity Research Information Centre (Association for the Study of Obesity): http://aso.org.uk
- Patient information: www.patient.co.uk
- Primary Care Society for Gastroenterology: www.pcsg.org.uk
- PRODIGY: near patient clinical support and patient information: www.prodigy.nhs.uk
- Royal College of General Practitioners: www.rcgp.org.uk
- Scottish Intercollegiate Guidelines Network (SIGN): www.sign.ac.uk
- The Obesity Awareness and Solutions Trust (TOAST): www.toast-uk.org
- Weight Concern: www.weightconcern.com
- Weight Wise (British Dietetic Association): www.bdaweightwise.com/bda

Useful journals
- *British Journal of General Practice*
- *British Medical Journal*
- *Gastroenterology* – official journal of the American Gastroenterology Association
- *GastroIMPACT* – newsletter aimed at GPs and associated healthcare professionals with an interest in gastrointestinal medicine (contact details: stuart@clynx.co.uk)
- *GUT* – official journal of the British Society of Gastroenterology
- *Lancet*
- *New England Journal of Medicine*

APPENDIX 2
Drugs commonly used in gastrointestinal practice

Drug/dose	Grouping	Disorder	Other information
Inflammatory bowel disease			
Azathioprine (2–2.5 mg/kg) 6-mercaptopurine (1–1.5 mg/kg)	Immuno-suppressant	Crohn's UC Autoimmune hepatitis	FBC, LFTs need monitoring weekly for 4 weeks, monthly for 2 months, then 1–3 monthly. Consider in UC/Crohn's if two courses of steroids within 1 year. Usual treatment duration is 3–4 years+ Appears to be safe to continue in pregnancy, but ideally do not start (see below) Side-effects: bone marrow suppression (5%), pancreatitis (2–3%), hypersensitivity Possible increase in incidence of lymphoma Takes 2–3 months to take effect
Methotrexate (im/sc) 25 mg ×1 per week for 16 weeks (induction of remission); 15mg ×1 per week for 40 weeks (? beyond) (maintenance)	Immuno-suppressant	Crohn's	FBC, LFTs monthly. Beware rare side-effect of interstitial pneumonitis (breathlessness) Teratogenic (men and premenopausal women *must* have efficient contraception and avoid pregnancy during and for 6 months after cessation of drug)

Drug/dose	Grouping	Disorder	Other information
Prednisolone (30–60 mg daily in tapering dose)	Immuno-suppressant	Crohn's UC Autoimmune hepatitis ?Alcoholic hepatitis	Usual to taper in UC by 5 mg/week; Crohn's often needs slower taper (e.g. 5 mg/fortnight) Consider concurrent bone protection (at least e.g. Calcichew D3 forte, but preferably a bisphosphonate) Prednisolone 30 mg daily for 1 month may improve prognosis in patients with alcoholic hepatitis, who have a high mortality
Budesonide (9 mg daily; 6 mg daily; 3 mg daily each dose for 1 month tapering)	Immuno-suppressant	Crohn's (ileocaecal) UC	More potent steroid, but with extensive first pass metabolism, therefore fewer side-effects For treatment of active disease; no role in maintenance
Infliximab (anti-TNF) (5 mg/kg as infusion) (induction and maintenance of remission)	Biological agent	Crohn's	Used in steroid-resistant/azathioprine/methotrexate-resistant/intolerant disease Highly effective (70–80% improve; 30% into remission) Concurrent azathioprine or methotrexate important as discourages formation of anti-TNF antibody formation (thus maintaining efficacy of infliximab)
Ciclosporin (2–4 mg/kg as infusion)	Immuno-suppressant	UC	Useful as 'rescue' therapy in severe UC not responding to iv hydrocortisone, with up to 80% responding;

Drug/dose	Grouping	Disorder	Other information
			however 50% will subsequently undergo colectomy in 1 year Consider particularly in first presentations and in those who are not on azathioprine
5-Aminosalicylates (5-ASAs)	5-Aminosali-cylates	UC ? Crohn's	Useful for the induction and maintenance of remission in UC (reduces risk of relapse two- to four-fold) Newer 5-ASAs no more effective than sulphasalazine, but fewer side-effects Minor effect in induction of remission in Crohn's (best evidence probably for Pentasa 4 g daily) Similar minor effect in maintenance of remission (6% ARR) – best evidence for maintenance in post-surgical group (13% ARR) May very rarely cause blood disorders (so warn about easy bruising, sore throats, etc.) Reports of interstitial nephritis – but very rare and no proven value to serial U&E tests
Sulfasalazine (1–2 g qds for active disease; 500 mg qds for maintenance)	5-Aminosali-cylate	UC ? Colonic Crohn's	May be particularly useful in patients with associated arthritides Causes reversible oligospermia
Mesalazine *Asacol*: 800 mg tds for active disease; 400–800 mg tds for maintenance	5-Aminosali-cylate	UC ? Colonic Crohn's	Different delivery systems exist: pH-dependent release in ileocaecal region (Asacol, Ipocol, Salofalk); slow release

Drug/dose	Grouping	Disorder	Other information
Pentasa: 3–4 g in divided doses for active disease; 2 g daily in divided doses for maintenance *Salofalk*: 500 mg tds for active disease; 250–500 mg tds for maintenance *Ipocol*: 800 mg tds for active disease; 400–800 mg tds for maintenance		? Colonic Crohn's	through ethylcellulose coating therefore releasing throughout small and large bowel (Pentasa) Higher doses are often used in USA Evidence suggests 3.6–4.8 g Asacol is more efficacious than standard dose in moderately severe UC. Mesalazine may be used as an enema, where it is at least as (if not more) efficacious as steroid enemas. Enemas are able to reach as far as the descending colon Suppositories are useful for proctitis
Balsalazide (2.25 g tds for active disease; 1.5 g bd for maintenance)	5-Aminosalicylate	UC ? Colonic Crohn's	5-ASA linked to a peptide (cleaved by colonic bacteria to release active 5-ASA)
Olsalazine (500 mg bd increasing to 1 g tds if necessary for active disease; 500 mg bd for maintenance	5-Aminosalicylate	UC ? Colonic Crohn's	Dimer of 5-ASA (azo bond cleaved by colonic bacteria) May cause diarrhoea, and therefore may be useful in distal colitis (often associated with proximal constipation)
Metronidazole (400 mg tds)	Antibiotic	Perianal Crohn's *Clostridium difficile* diarrhoea	First line agent for *C. difficile* diarrhoea Useful in perianal Crohn's Beware peripheral neuropathy No alcohol (antabuse-like reaction)

Drug/dose	Grouping	Disorder	Other information
			Evidence suggests 20 mg/kg/day for 3 months after ileal resection delays Crohn's recurrence
Vancomycin (125 mg qds oral)	Antibiotic	*Clostridium difficile* diarrhoea	Alternative agent for *C. difficile* diarrhoea
Elemental 028	Elemental nutrition	Crohn's (particularly small bowel disease)	Useful in the treatment of small bowel Crohn's disease, especially where possible side-effects of steroids are particularly undesirable (e.g. adolescents, osteoporotic vertebral collapse)
Irritable bowel syndrome			
Isphagula husk (Fybogel/Regulan) (1–3 sachets daily)	Bulking agent/ laxative	IBS Constipation	Proven value in IBS
Peppermint oil (1 capsule tds)	Smooth muscle relaxant	IBS	May be tried as there is evidence of effect in individual trials, but meta-analysis shows no difference compared to placebo
Mebeverine (Colofac) (135 mg tds)	Smooth muscle relaxant	IBS	Global improvement in symptoms but no effect on pain
Alverine citrate (Spasmonal) (60–120 mg tds)	Smooth muscle relaxant	IBS	
Cimetropium bromide	Smooth muscle relaxant	IBS	Good for pain in IBS (not available in the UK)
Dicyclomine bromide (Merbentyl) (10–20 mg tds)	Antimuscarinic (anticholinergic)	IBS	Good for pain in IBS
Amitriptyline (10–75 mg nocte)	Tricyclic antidepressant	IBS/ coexistent depression	Start low-dose at night-time 10–25mg Good evidence for efficacy in relief of pain

Drug/dose	Grouping	Disorder	Other information
			Constipating side-effect makes it particularly useful in diarrhoea-predominant IBS Other tricyclics may be used: tramipramine, desipramine, clomipramine
Fluoxetine/ citalopram (20 mg od)	Selective serotonin re-uptake inhibitors	IBS	Increasingly used in IBS but no published randomised controlled trials in IBS. Diarrhoea side-effect, therefore consider in constipation-predominant IBS
Alosetron	5HT$_3$-receptor antagonist	IBS	Restricted use in USA (not available UK) Useful in relieving pain and diarrhoea in female diarrhoea-predominant IBS, but withdrawn over concerns of an association with ischaemic colitis
Tegaserod	5HT$_4$-receptor partial agonist	IBS	Small beneficial effect in (female) constipation-predominant IBS
Constipation			
Isphagula husk (Fybogel, Isogel, Ispagel, Konsyl. Regulan) (1-3 sachets daily)	Bulking laxative	Constipation IBS	See above (in IBS) Bulking agents may also help in chronic diarrhoea
Methylcellulose (Celevac) (3–6 tablets bd)	Bulking laxative	Constipation	As above
Sterculia (Normacol) (1–2 sachets od/bd)	Bulking laxative	Constipation	As above
Bisacodyl (5–10 mg nocte, increasing to 15–20 mg if required)	Stimulant laxative (also as suppository)	Constipation	Chronic use of stimulant laxatives may precipitate onset of an atonic, non-functioning colon

Drug/dose	Grouping	Disorder	Other information
Docusate sodium (up to 500 mg/day in divided doses)	Stimulant (and softening) laxative Also as enema (e.g. Fletchers enemette)	Constipation	As above
Senna (Senna, Manevac) (2–4 tablets nocte)	Stimulant laxative	Constipation	May cause cramps (also see above under bisacodyl)
Glycerol suppositories	Stimulant/irritative	Constipation	
Lactulose (10–20 ml bd)	Osmotic laxative	Constipation Hepatic enceph-alopathy	Results in an acidic diarrhoea (low pH) which is useful in the treatment of hepatic encephalopathy (discourages proliferation of ammonia-producing organisms) May cause abdominal cramps and flatulence
Liquid paraffin	Osmotic laxative	Constipation	Not recommended Problems with anal seepage, granulomatous reactions, lipoid pneumonia if aspirated, and may interfere with absorption of vitamins A, D, E, K (fat soluble)
Macrogols (Idrolax, Movicol) (1–3 sachets daily)	Osmotic laxative	Constipation	Holds onto administered water May cause abdominal pain and distension
Phosphate enema (Fleet ready-to-use-enema, Fletchers' phosphate enema)	Osmotic laxative	Constipation Bowel preparation	Often used to clear distal bowel prior to flexible sigmoidoscopy

Drug/dose	Grouping	Disorder	Other information
Obesity			
Orlistat (120 mg immediately before, during, or <1 hour after main meal; max 360 mg daily)	Lipase inhibitor	Obesity	See NICE guidelines 2001 (update expected 2006) May cause steatorrhoea and diminish vitamin D levels, anal seepage. NICE (2001) recommended: 'Only treat those who lose >2.5 kg by diet/exercise in the preceding month, and for >3 months if weight loss >5%; >6 months if weight loss >10% baseline. Treatment normally ceases at 1 year; *never beyond 2 years.'* This guidance is under review and advice in the *British National Formulary* (September 2005) suggests an anti-obesity drug should be considered only for those who have received at least 3 months of managed care involving a supervised diet, exercise and behaviour modification who have failed to achieve a realistic reduction in weight. In the presence of risk factors (such as diabetes, coronary heart disease, hypertension, and obstructive sleep apnoea), it may be appropriate to prescribe a drug to individuals with a BMI of 27 kg/m^2 (as opposed to usual

Drug/dose	Grouping	Disorder	Other information
			value: 30 kg/m^2) or greater. The individual should be monitored on a regular basis. Drug treatment should be discontinued if weight loss is less than 5% after the first 12 weeks or if the individual regains weight at any time while receiving drug treatment
Sibutramine (10 mg, increasing to 15 mg after 1 month if weight loss <2 kg)	Centrally acting appetite suppressant	Obesity	See NICE guidelines and comments above

ARR, absolute risk reduction; bd, twice a day; BMI, body mass index; FBC, full blood count; IBS, inflammatory bowel disease; im, intramuscular; iv, intravenous; LFTs, liver function tests; nocte, at night; od, once a day; qds, four times a day; tds, three times a day; TNF, tumour necrosis factor; sc, subcutaneous; UC, ulcerative colitis; U&E, urea and electrolytes.

REFERENCES

CHAPTER 1

Devesa SS, Blot WJ, Fraumeni JF Jr. Changing patterns in the incidence of esophageal and gastric cardiac carcinoma in the United States. Cancer 1998; 83: 2049–2053

Kelsen DP, Ginsberg R, Pajak TF et al. Chemotherapy followed by surgery compared with surgery alone for localized oesophageal cancer. N Engl J Med 1998; 339(27): 1979–1984

Lagegren J, Bergstrom R, Lingren A, Nyren O. Symptomatic gastroesophageal reflux as a risk factor for esophageal adenocarcinoma. N Engl J Med 1999; 340: 333–340

Wychulis AR, Woolman G, Andersen HA, Ellis FH Jr. Achalasia and carcinoma of the oesophagus. JAMA 1981; 125: 1638

CHAPTER 2

Castell DO, Kahrilas PJ, Richter JE et al. Esomeprazole (40mg) compared with lansoprazole (30mg) in the treatment of erosive esophagitis. Am J Gastroenterol 2002; 97: 575–583

Christie J, Shepherd NA, Codling BW, Valori RM. Gastric cancer below the age of 55: implications for screening patients with uncomplicated dyspepsia. Gut 1997; 41: 513–517

Danesh J, Lawrence M, Murphy M, Roberts S, Collins R. A systematic review of the epidemiological evidence on Helicobacter pylori and nonulcer or uninvestigated dyspepsia. Arch Intern Med 2000; 160: 1192–1198

Drugs and Therapeutics Bulletin. Should H. pylori be eradicated in non-ulcer dyspepsia? DTB 2002; 40(3): 23–24

Jaakkimainen RL, Boyle E, Tudiver F. Is Helicobacter pylori associated with non-ulcer dyspepsia and will eradication improve symptoms? A meta-analysis. BMJ 1999; 319: 1040–1044

Joelsson B, Johnsson F. Heartburn – the acid test. Gut 1989; 30: 1523–1525

Kuipers EJ, Lundell L, Klinkenberg-Knol EC et al. Atrophic gastritis and Helicobacter pylori infection in patients with reflux oesophagitis treated with omeprazole or fundoplication. N Engl J Med 1996; 334: 1018–1022

Lagergren J, Bergstom R, Lindgren A, Nyren O. Symptomatic gastroesophageal reflux as a risk factor for esophageal adenocarcinoma. N Engl J Med 1999; 340: 825–831

Laine L, Schoenfeld P, Fennerty MB. Therapy for Helicobacter pylori in patients with nonulcer dyspepsia. Ann Intern Med 2001; 134: 361–369

Lauritsen K, Deviere J, Bigard MA et al. Esomeprazole 20mg and lansoprazole 15mg in maintaining healed reflux oesophagitis: Metropole study results. Aliment Pharmacol Ther 2003; 17: 333–341

Lundell L, Miettinen P, Myrvold HE et al. Lack of effect of acid suppression therapy on gastric atrophy: Nordic GERD Study Group. Gastroenterology 1999; 117: 319–326

McColl KEL, El-Nujumi A, Murray I et al. The H. pylori breath test: a surrogate marker for peptic ulcer disease in dyspeptic patients. Gut 1997; 40: 302–306

Moayyedi P, Soo S, Deeks J, Innes MA, Forman D, Delaney BC. A systematic review and economic analysis of the cost effectiveness of H. pylori eradication therapy in non-ulcer dyspepsia patients. BMJ 2000; 321: 659–664

Moayyedi P, Soo S, Deeks J et al. *Helicobacter pylori* eradication does not exacerbate reflux symptoms in gastroesophageal reflux disease. Gastroenterology 2001; 121: 1120–1126

National Institute for Health and Clinical Excellence (NICE). Dyspepsia: managing dyspepsia in adults in primary care. Quick reference guide. 2004. Online. Available: www.nice.org.uk/CG017

Nyren O, Adami HO, Bates S et al. Absence of therapeutic benefit from antacids or cimetidine in non-ulcer dyspepsia. N Engl J Med 1986; 314: 339–343

Sloan S, Rademaker AW, Kahrilas PJ. Determinants of gastroesophageal junction incompetence: hiatus hernia, lower esophageal sphincter, or both? Ann Intern Med 1992; 117: 977–982

Tally NJ, Colin-Jones D, Koch KJ et al. Functional dyspepsia: a classification with guidelines for diagnosis and management. Gastroenterol Int 1991; 4: 145–160

Tally NJ, Silverstein MD, Agreus I, Nyren O, Sonnenberg A, Holtmann G. American Gastroenterological Association technical review: evaluation of dyspepsia. Gastroenterology 1998a; 114: 582–595

Tally NJ, Meineche-Schmidt V, Pare P et al. Efficacy of omeprazole in functional dyspepsia: double-blind, randomized placebo-controlled trials (the Bond and Opera studies). Aliment Pharmacol Ther 1998b; 12: 1055–1065

Tally NJ, Stanghellini V, Heading RC et al. Functional gastroduodenal disorders. Gut 1999; 45(Suppl II): 1137–1142

CHAPTER 3

Lai BS, Kwong KH, Leung KL et al. Randomized trial of early vs delayed laparoscopic cholecystectomy for acute cholecystitis. Br J Surg 1998; 85: 767–770

Lo CM, Liu CL, Fan ST et al. Prospective randomised study of early vs delayed laparoscopic cholecystectomy for acute cholecystitis. Ann Surg 1998; 227: 461–467

Papi C, Catarci M, D'Ambrosio L et al. Timing of cholecystectomy for acute calculus cholecystitis: a meta-analysis. Am J Gastroenterol 2004; 99: 147–155

Steinberg W, Tenner S. Acute pancreatitis. N Engl J Med 1994; 330: 1198–1209

CHAPTER 4

Bacon BR, Faravash MJ, Janney CG et al. Non-alcoholic steatohepatitis: an expanded clinical entity. Gastroenterology 1994; 107: 1103–1106

Chalasani N, Aliadhey H, Kesterson J, Murray MD, Hall SD. Patients with elevated liver enzymes are not at higher risk for statin hepatotoxicity. Gastroenterology 2004; 126: 1287–1292 (see also Editorial, pp 1477–1479)

Cohen JA, Kaplan MM. The SGOT/SGPT ratio – an indicator of alcoholic liver disease. Dig Dis Sci 1979; 24: 835–838

Di Marco V, Lo Iacono O, Camma C et al. The long term course of chronic hepatitis B. Hepatology 1999; 30(1): 257–264

Goulis J, Leandro G, Burroughs A. Randomised controlled trials of ursodeoxycholic acid therapy for primary biliary cirrhosis: a meta-analysis. Lancet 1999; 354: 1053–1060

Matteoni C, Younossi ZM, Gramlich T et al. Nonalcoholic fatty liver disease: a spectrum of clinical pathological severity. Gastroenterology 1999; 116: 1413–1419

Pratt DS, Kaplan MM. Primary care: evaluation of abnormal liver-enzyme results in asymptomatic patients. N Engl J Med 2000; 342: 1266–1271

Roberts SK, Therneau T, Czaja AJ. Prognosis of histological cirrhosis in type 1 autoimmune hepatitis. Gastroenterology 1996; 110: 848–857

Skelly MM, James PD, Ryder SD. Findings on liver biopsy to investigate abnormal liver function tests in the absence of diagnostic serology. J Hepatol 2001; 35: 195–199

Weissberg J, Andres L, Smith C et al. Survival in chronic hepatitis B: an analysis of 379 patients. Ann Intern Med 1984; 101: 613–616

CHAPTER 5

Bampton PA, Holloway RH. A prospective study of the gastroenterological causes of iron deficiency anaemia in a General Hospital. Aust NZ J Med 1996; 26: 793–799

Bini EJ, Micale PL, Weinshel EH. Evaluation of the gastrointestinal tract in premenopausal women with iron deficiency anaemia [see comments]. Am J Med 1998; 105: 281–286

Cook IJ, Pavli P, Riley JW et al. Gastrointestinal investigation of iron deficiency anaemia. Br Med J 1986; 292: 1380–1382

Goddard AF, James MW, McIntyre AS et al. Guidelines for the management of iron deficiency anaemia. British Society of Gastroenterology: June 2000, updated May 2005. Online. Available: www.bsg.org.uk

Green BT, Rockey DC. Gastrointestinal endoscopic evaluation of pre-menopausal women with iron deficiency anaemia. J Clin Gastroenterol 2004; 38: 104–109

Hardwick RH, Armstrong CP. Synchronous upper and lower gastrointestinal endoscopy is an effective method of investigating iron-deficiency anaemia. Br J Surg 1997; 84: 1725–1728

Ioannou GN, Rockey DC, Bryson CL et al. Iron deficiency and gastrointestinal malignancy: a population-based cohort study. Am J Med 2003; 113: 276–280

Joosten E, Dereymaeker L, Pelemans W, Hiele M. Significance of a low serum ferritin level in elderly in-patients. Postgrad Med J 1993; 69: 397–400

Joosten E, Ghesquiere B, Linthoudt H et al. Upper and lower gastrointestinal evaluation of elderly inpatients who are iron deficient. Am J Med 1999; 107: 24–29

Kepczyk T, Kadakia SC. Prospective evaluation of gastrointestinal tract in patients with iron deficiency anaemia. Dig Dis Sci 1995; 40: 1283–1289

Kepczyk T, Cremins JE, Long BD, Bachinski BZ, Smith RL, McNally PR. A prospective, multidisciplinary evaluation of premenopausal women with iron-deficiency anaemia. Am J Gastroenterol 1999; 94: 109–115

Kerlin P, Reiner R, Davies M, Sage RE, Grant AK. Iron deficiency anaemia – a prospective study. Aust NZ J Med 1979; 9: 402–417

Lee JG, Sahagun G, Oehlke M, Liebermann DA. Serious gastrointestinal pathology found in patients with serum ferritin values <50 ng/ml. Am J Gastroenterol 1998; 93: 772–776

McIntyre AS, Long RG. Prospective survey of investigations in outpatients referred with iron deficiency anaemia. Gut 1993; 34: 1102–1107

Rockey DC, Cello JP. Evaluation of the gastrointestinal tract in patients with iron deficiency anaemia. N Engl J Med 1993; 329: 1691–1695

Sahay R, Scott BB. Iron deficiency anaemia – how far to investigate? Gut 1993; 34: 1427–1428

CHAPTER 6

Akehurst R, Kaltenthaler E. Treatment of irritable bowel syndrome: a review of randomised controlled trials. Gut 2001; 48(2): 272–282

Camilleri M, Northcutt AR, Kong S, Dukes GE, McSorley D, Mangel AW. Efficacy and safety of alosetron in women with irritable bowel syndrome: a randomised, placebo-controlled trial. Lancet 2000; 355: 1035–1040

Drossman DA, Li Z, Andruzzi E et al. U.S. Householder Survey of functional gastrointestinal disorders: prevalence, sociodemography and health impact. Dig Dis Sci 1993; 38: 1569–1580

Drugs and Therapeutics Bulletin. Hypnotherapy for functional gastrointestinal disorders. DTB 2005; 43: 45–48

Gwee KA, Leong YL, Graham C et al. The role of psychological and biological factors in postinfective gut dysfunction. Gut 1999; 44: 400–406

Hamm LR, Sorrells SC, Harding JP et al. Additional investigations fail to alter the diagnosis of irritable bowel syndrome in subjects fulfilling the Rome criteria. Am J Gastroenterol 1999; 94: 1279–1282

Jackson JL, O'Malley PG, Tomkins G et al. Treatment of functional gastrointestinal disorders with antidepressant medications: a meta-analysis. Am J Med 2000; 108: 65–72

McKendrick MW, Read NW. Irritable bowel syndrome – post salmonella infection. J Infect 1994; 29: 1–3

Mueller-Lissner S, Fumagalli I, Bardhan KD et al. Tegaserod, a 5-HT4 receptor partial agonist, relieves key symptoms of irritable bowel syndrome [abstract]. Gastroenterology 2000; 118: A175

Nanda R, James R, Smith H et al. Food intolerance and the irritable bowel syndrome. Gut 1989; 30: 1099–1104

Pittler MH, Ernst E. Peppermint oil for irritable bowel syndrome: a critical review and metaanalysis. Am J Gastroenterol 1998; 93: 1131–1135

Poynard T, Naveau S, Mory B et al. Meta-analysis of smooth muscle relaxants in the treatment of irritable bowel syndrome. Aliment Pharmacol Ther 1994; 8: 499–510

Prior A, Whorwell PJ. Double blind study of ispaghula in irritable bowel syndrome. Gut 1987; 28: 1510–1513

Rodriguez LA, Ruigomez A. Increased risk of irritable bowel syndrome after bacterial gastroenteritis. BMJ 1999; 318: 565–566

Sanders DS, Carter MJ, Hurlstone DP et al. Association of adult coeliac disease with irritable bowel syndrome: a case-control study in patients fulfilling the Rome II criteria referred to secondary care. Lancet 2001; 358: 1504–1508

Snook J, Shepherd HA. Bran supplementation in the treatment of irritable bowel syndrome. Aliment Pharmacol Ther 1994; 8: 511–514

Vanner SJ, Depew WT, Paterson W et al. Predictive value of the Rome criteria for diagnosing the irritable bowel syndrome. Am J Gastroenterol 1999; 94: 2912–2917

Whorwell PJ, Prior A, Faragher EB. Controlled trial of hypnotherapy in the treatment of severe refractory irritable bowel syndrome. Lancet 1984; 2: 1232–1234

Whorwell PJ, Prior A, Colgan SM. Hypnotherapy in severe irritable bowel syndrome: further experience. Gut 1987; 28: 423–425

CHAPTER 7

Attar A, Lemann M, Ferguson A et al. Comparison of a low-dose polyethylene glycol-electrolyte solution with lactulose for treatment of chronic constipation. Gut 1999; 44: 226–230

Burkitt DP, Walker ARP, Painter NS. Effect of dietary fibre on stools and transit times and its role in the causation of disease. Lancet 1972; ii: 1408–1412

Department of Health. Prescription cost analysis: England 2001. Online. Available: www.dh.gov.uk/Publications AndStatistics/Statistics/StatisticalWork Areas/StatisticalHealthCare/Statistical HealthCareArticle/fs/en?CONTENT_ID= 4015540&chk=P%2BZ80%2B

Frizelle F, Barclay M. Constipation in adults. In: Clinical Evidence 2004. Online.

Available: www.clinicalevidence.com/ceweb/conditions/dsd/0413/0413_background.jsp

Prather CM, Camilleri M, Zinsmeister AR et al. Tegaserod accelerates orocecal transit in patients with constipation-predominant irritable bowel syndrome. Gastroenterology 2000; 118: 463–468

Thompson WG, Heaton KW. Functional bowel disorders in apparently healthy people. Gastroenterology 1980; 79: 283–288

CHAPTER 8

Camma C, Giunta M, Rosselli M et al. Mesalamine in the maintenance treatment of Crohn's disease: a meta-analysis adjusted for confounding variables. Gastroenterology 1997; 113: 1465–1473

Feagan BG, Rochon J, Fedorak RN et al. Methotrexate for the treatment of Crohn's disease. N Engl J Med 1995; 332: 292–297

Feagan BG, Fedorak RN, Irvine EJ et al. A comparison of methotrexate with placebo for the maintenance of remission in Crohn's disease. N Engl J Med 2000; 342: 1627–1632

Jones J, Boorman J, Cann P et al. British Society of Gastroenterology guidelines for the management of the irritable bowel syndrome. Gut 2000; (Suppl II)47: ii1–ii19

Lichtiger S, Present DH, Kornbluth A. Cyclosporin in severe ulcerative colitis refractory to steroid therapy. N Engl J Med 1994; 330: 1841–1845

Lochs H, Mayer M, Fleig WE et al. Prophylaxis of postoperative relapse in Crohn's disease with mesalazine: European Cooperative Crohn's Disease Study VI. Gastroenterology 2000; 118: 264–273

Mekhjian HS, Switz DM, Watts HD et al. National Co-operative Crohn's Disease Study: factors determining recurrence of Crohn's disease after surgery. Gastroenterology 1979; 77: 907–913

Robinson A, Thompson DG, Wilkin D et al. Guided self-management and practice-directed follow-up of ulcerative colitis: a randomised trial. Lancet 2001; 358: 976–981

Singleton JW, Hanauer SB, Gitnick GL et al. Mesalamine capsules for the treatment of active Crohn's disease: results of a 16-week trial. Pentasa Crohn's Disease Study Group. Gastroenterology 1993; 104: 1293–1301

Targan SR, Hanauer SB, von Deventer SJ et al. A short-term study of chimeric monoclonal antibody cA2 to tumor necrosis factor alpha for Crohn's disease. Crohn's Disease cA2 Study Group. N Engl J Med 1997; 337: 1029–1035

Truelove SC, Witts LJ. Cortisone in ulcerative colitis – final report on a therapeutic trial. BMJ 1955; 2: 1041–1048

CHAPTER 9

Crossland, A, Jones , R. Rectal bleeding; prevalence and consultation behaviour. BMJ 1995; 311: 486–488

Department of Health. Guidance on commissioning cancer services: improving outcomes in colorectal cancer. Department of Health, Clinical Outcomes Group, Cancer Guidance sub-group. 1997. Department of Health, London

Flashman K, O'Leary DP, Senapati A, Thompson, MR. The Department of Health's 'two week standard' for bowel cancer: is it working? Gut 2004; 53: 387–391

Jonas M, Schofield J. Anal fissure (chronic). In: Clinical Evidence 2004. Online. Available: www.clinicalevidence.com/ceweb/conditions/dsd/0407/0407_I2.jsp

Simpson J, Spiller R. Colonic diverticular disease. In: Clinical Evidence 2004. Online. Available: www.clinical

evidence.com/ceweb/conditions/dsd/
0405/0405.jsp

Thompson MR, Heath I, Ellis BG et al.
Identifying and managing patients at
low risk of bowel cancer in general
practice. BMJ 2003; 327: 263–265

CHAPTER 11

British National Formulary, 49th edn. 2005.
Online. Available: www.bnf.org

Flegal KM, Carroll MD, Ogden CL, Johnson
CL. Prevalence and trends in obesity
among US adults, 1999-2000. JAMA
2002; 288: 1723–1727

Heymsfield SB, Greenberg AS, Fujioka K
et al. Recombinant leptin for weight loss
in obese and lean adults: a randomised,
controlled, dose-escalation trial. JAMA
1999; 282: 1568–1575

National Heart, Lung and Blood Institute.
Clinical guidelines on the identification,
evaluation, and treatment of overweight
and obesity in adults – the evidence
report. Obes Res 1998; 6(Suppl 2):
51S–209S

National Institute for Clinical Excellence.
NICE issues guidance on orlistat for
obesity. 2001. Online. Available:
www.nice.org.uk/page.aspx?o=37995

Nicholson FB, Korman MG, Richardson
MA. Percutaneous endoscopic
gastrostomy: a review of indications,
complications and outcome.
J Gastroenterol Hepatol 2000; 15: 21–25

Office for National Statistics. Body mass: by
sex, 2001. Social Trends 33 (updated
29.1.03)

CHAPTER 12

Allison JE, Tekawa IS, Ransom LJ, Adrian
AL. A comparison of fecal occult-blood
tests for colorectal-cancer screening.
N Engl J Med 1996; 334: 155–159

Atkin WS, Northover JM. Protagonist:
population based endoscopic screening
for colorectal cancer. Gut 2003; 52:
321–322

Byers T, Levin B, Rothenberger D et al.
American Cancer Society guidelines for
screening and surveillance for early
detection of colorectal polyps and
cancer: Update 1997. CA Cancer J Clin
1997; 47: 154–160

Cairns S, Scholefield JH (eds) Guidelines for
colorectal cancer screening in high risk
groups. Gut 2002; 51(Suppl IV): v1–v29

Cameron AJ, Lomboy CT, Pera M et al.
Adenocarcinoma of the esophagogastric
junction and Barrett's oesophagus.
Gastroenterology 1995; 109(5): 1541–1546

Cullen KJ, Stevens DP, Frost MA, Mackay
IR. Carcinoembryonic antigen (CEA),
smoking, and cancer in a longitudinal
population study. Aust N Z J Med 1976;
6: 279–283

Gondal G, Grotmal T, Hofstad B et al.
Grading of distal colorectal adenomas as
predictors for proximal neoplasia and
choice of endoscope in population
screening: experience from the
Norwegian Colorectal Cancer
Prevention study (NORCCAP) Gut
2003; 52: 398–403

Hardcastle JD, Chamberlain JO, Robinson
MHE et al. Randomised controlled trial
of faecal-occult-blood screening for
colorectal cancer. Lancet 1996; 348:
1472–1477

Hine KR, Booth SN, Leonard JC, Dykes PW.
Carcinoembryonic antigen
concentrations in undiagnosed patients.
Lancet 1978; 2: 1337–1340

Johnson PJ, Portmann B, Williams R.
Alpha-fetoprotein concentrations
measured by radioimmunoassay in
diagnosing and excluding hepatocellular
carcinoma. Br Med J 1978; 2: 661–663

Liaw YF, Tai DI, Chu CM et al. Early
detection of hepatocellular carcinoma in
patients with chronic type B hepatitis. A
prospective study. Gastroenterology
1986; 90: 263–267

Macafee DA, Scholefield JH. Antagonist:
population based endoscopic screening

for colorectal cancer. Gut 2003; 52: 323–326

Macrae F, St John DJ. Relationship between patterns of bleeding and haemoccult sensitivity in patients with colorectal cancers or adenomas. Gastroenterology 1982; 82: 891–898

Mandel JS, Bond JH, Church TR et al. Reducing mortality from colorectal cancer by screening for fecal occult blood. N Engl J Med 1993; 328: 1365–1371

Maringhini A, Cottone M, Sciarrino E et al. Ultrasonography and alpha-fetoprotein in diagnosis of hepatocellular carcinoma in cirrhosis. Dig Dis Sci 1988; 33: 47–51

Muller AD, Sonnenberg A. Prevention of colorectal cancer by flexible endoscopy and polypectomy. A case-control study of 32,702 veterans. Ann Intern Med 1995; 123: 904–910

Oka H, Kurioka N, Kim K et al. Prospective study of early detection of hepatocellular carcinoma in patients with cirrhosis. Hepatology 1990; 12: 680–687

Piantino P, Andriulli A, Gindro T et al. CA19-9 assay in differential diagnosis of pancreatic carcinoma from inflammatory pancreatic diseases. Am J Gastroenterol 1986; 81: 436–439

Pleskow DK, Berger HJ, Gyves J, Allen E, McLean A, Podolsky DK. Evaluation of a serological marker, CA19-9, in the diagnosis of pancreatic cancer. Ann Intern Med 1989; 110: 704–709

Ryder SD. Guidelines for the diagnosis and treatment of hepatocellular carcinoma. Gut 2003; 52(Suppl III): iii1–iii8

Selby JV, Friedman GD, Quesenberry CP et al. A case-control study of screening sigmoidoscopy and mortality from colorectal cancer. N Engl J Med 1992; 326: 653–657

Steinberg W. The clinical utility of the CA19-9 tumor-associated antigen. Am J Gastroenterol 1990; 85: 350–355

Steinberg WM, Gelfand R, Anderson KK et al. Comparison of the sensitivity and specificity of the CA19-9 and carcinoembryonic antigen assays in detecting cancer of the pancreas. Gastroenterology 1986; 90: 343–349

Tang ZY, Yu YQ, Zhou XD, Yang BH, Ma ZC, Lin ZY. Subclinical hepatocellular carcinoma: an analysis of 391 patients. J Surg Oncol 1993; 3(Suppl): 55–58

Towler BP, Irwig L, Glasziou P et al. Screening for colorectal cancer using the faecal occult blood test, Hemoccult (Cochrane Review). In: The Cochrane Library, Issue 3, 1998. Oxford: Update Software

van den Burgh, Dees J, Hop WCJ et al. Oesophageal cancer is an uncommon cause of death in patients with Barrett's oesophagus. Gut 1996; 39: 5–9

Wanebo HJ, Rao B, Pinsky CM et al. Preoperative carcinoembryonic antigen level as a prognostic indicator in colorectal cancer. N Engl J Med 1978; 299: 448–451

Winawer SJ, Zauber AG, Ho MN et al. Prevention of colorectal cancer by colonoscopic polypectomy. The National Polyp Study Workgroup. N Engl J Med 1993; 329: 1977–1981

Winawer SJ, Fletcher RH, Miller L et al. Colorectal cancer screening: clinical guidelines and rationale. Gastroenterology 1997; 112: 594–642

Wright TA, Gray MR, Morris AI et al. Cost effectiveness of detecting Barrett's cancer. Gut 1996; 39(4): 574–579

CHAPTER 13

Bowles CJ, Leicester R, Romaya C et al. A prospective study of colonoscopy practice in the UK today: are we adequately prepared for national colorectal cancer screening tomorrow? Gut 2004; 53: 277–283

Johnson CD, Harmsen WS, Wilson LA et al. Prospective blinded evaluation of computed tomographic colonography for screen detection of colorectal polyps. Gastroenterology 2003; 125: 311–319

Pineau BC, Paskett ED, Chen GJ et al. Virtual colonoscopy using oral contrast compared with colonoscopy for the detection of patients with colorectal polyps. Gastroenterology 2003; 125: 304–310

Rex DK. Is virtual colonoscopy ready for widespread application? Gastroenterology 2003; 125: 608–610

Rex DK, Rahmani EY, Haseman JH et al. Relative sensitivity of colonoscopy and barium enema for detection of colorectal cancer in clinical practice. Gastroenterology 1997a; 112: 17–23

Rex DK, Cutler CS, Lemmel GT et al. Colonoscopic miss rates of adenomas determined by back-to-back colonoscopies. Gastroenterology 1997b; 112: 24–28

Winawer SJ, Stewart ET, Zauber AG et al. A comparison of colonoscopy and double-contrast barium enema for surveillance after polypectomy. N Engl J Med 2000; 342: 1766–1772

CHAPTER 14

Alstead EM, Nelson-Piercy C. Inflammatory bowel disease in pregnancy. Gut 2003; 52: 159–161

Carter MJ, Lobo AJ, Travis SPL. Guidelines for the management of inflammatory bowel disease in adults. Gut 2004; 53(Suppl V): v1–v16

D'Amico G, Pagliaro L, Bosch J. Pharmacological treatment of portal hypertension; an evidence-based approach. Semin Liver Dis 1999; 19: 475–505

Feagan BG, Fedorak RN, Irvine EJ et al. A comparison of methotrexate with placebo for the maintenance of remission in Crohn's disease. N Engl J Med 2000; 342: 1627–1632

Feagan BG, Rochon J, Fedorak RN et al. Methotrexate for the treatment of Crohn's disease. N Engl J Med 1995; 332: 292–297

Francella A, Dyan A, Bodian C et al. The safety of 6-mercaptopurine for child-bearing patients with inflammatory bowel disease: a retrospective cohort study. Gastroenterology 2003; 124: 9–17

Goulis J, Leandro G, Burroughs AK. Randomised controlled trials of ursodeoxycholic acid therapy for primary biliary cirrhosis. Lancet 1999; 354: 1053–1060

Jalan R, Hayes P. UK guidelines on the management of variceal haemorrhage in cirrhotic patients. Gut 2000; 46(Suppl III): iii1–iii15

Lennard L. TPMT in the treatment of Crohn's disease with azathioprine. Gut 2002; 51: 143–146

Lichtiger S, Present DH, Kornbluth A. Cylcosporin in severe ulcerative colitis refractory to steroid therapy. N Engl J Med 1994; 330: 1841–1845

Lofberg R, Danielsson A, Suhr O et al. Oral budesonide versus prednisolone in patients with active extensive and left sided colitis. Gastroenterology 1996; 110: 1713–1718.

May GR, Sutherland GR, Shaffer EA. Efficacy of bile acid therapy for gallstone dissolution: a meta-analysis of randomised trials. Aliment Pharmacol Ther 1993; 7: 139–148

National Institute for Health and Clinical Excellence (NICE). NICE issues guidance on proton pump inhibitors (PPI) for dyspepsia. 2000. Online. Available: www.nice.org.uk/page. aspx?o=38034

National Institute for Health and Clinical Excellence (NICE). NICE issues guidance on orlistat for obesity. 2001. Online. Available: www.nice.org.uk/page.aspx?o=37995

Norgard B, Fonager K, Pedersen L et al. Birth outcome in women exposed to 5-aminosalicylic acid during pregnancy:

a Danish cohort study. Gut 2003; 52: 243–247

Poupon R, Lindor KD, Cauch-Dudek K et al. Combined analysis of French, American and Canadian randomised controlled trials of ursodeoxycholic acid therapy in primary biliary cirrhosis. Gastroenterology 1997; 113: 884–890

Poynard T, Cales P, Pasta L, et al. Beta-adrenergic-antagonist drugs in the prevention of gastrointestinal bleeding in patients with cirrhosis and esophageal varices: an analysis of data and prognostic factors in 589 patients from four randomized clinical trials. N Engl J Med 1991; 324: 1532–1538

Present DH, Rutgeerts P, Targan S et al. Infliximab for the treatment of fistulas in patients with Crohn's disease. N Engl J Med 1999; 340: 1398–1405

Rutgeerts P, Lofberg R, Malchow H et al. A comparison of budesonide with prednisolone for active Crohn's disease. N Engl J Med 1994; 331: 842–845.

Targan SR, Hanauer SB, van Deventer SJ et al. A short term study of chimeric monoclonal antibody cA2 to tumour necrosis factor alpha for Crohn's disease. Crohn's disease cA2 Study Group. N Engl J Med 1997; 337: 1029–1035

CHAPTER 15

Allum WH, Griffin SM, Watson A et al. Guidelines for the management of oesophageal and gastric cancer. British Society of Gastroenterology, May 2002. Online. Available: www.bsg.org.uk/pdf_word_docs/ogcancer.pdf

Herskovic A, Martz K, Al Sarraf M et al. Combined chemotherapy and radiotherapy compared with radiotherapy alone in patients with cancer of the oesophagus. N Engl J Med 1992; 326: 1593–1598

Meyerhardt JA, Mayer RJ. Systemic therapy for colorectal cancer. N Engl J Med 2005; 352: 476–487

Ryder SD. Guidelines for the diagnosis and treatment of hepatocellular carcinoma (HCC) in adults. Gut 2003; 52(Suppl III): iii1–iii8

LIST OF PATIENT QUESTIONS

INDEX

Page numbers in **bold** refer to boxes, figures and tables

D